TM 8-225

WAR DEPARTMENT
TECHNICAL MANUAL

DENTAL TECHNICIANS

January 28, 1942

TECHNICAL MANUAL
No. 8-225

WAR DEPARTMENT,
WASHINGTON, January 28, 1942.

TM 8-225

DENTAL TECHNICIANS

Prepared under direction of
The Surgeon General

	Paragraphs
CHAPTER 1. General	1
CHAPTER 2. Mouth and teeth.	
SECTION I. General	2-3
II. Teeth	4-7
III. Regional anatomy	8-14
IV. Definitions	15
CHAPTER 3. Prosthetic technician.	
SECTION I. General	16
II. Impression materials	17
III. Plaster impressions	18-22
IV. Modeling compound impressions	23-25
V. Hydrocolloid impressions	26
VI. Construction of full and partial vulcanite dentures	27-48
VII. Acrylic resin dentures	49-50
VIII. Denture repair	51-58
IX. Dental castings	59-62
X. Cast crowns	63-65
XI. Cast occlusal gold crown	66-67
XII. Fixed bridge	68-71
XIII. Clasps and bars for partial dentures	72-78
XIV. Cast partial dentures and partial denture skeletons	79-93
XV. Splints	94-97
CHAPTER 4. Dental X-ray technician.	
SECTION I. Equipment	98-103
II. Intra-oral roentgenography	104-125
III. Extra-oral roentgenography	126-129
IV. Processing of X-ray films	130-138
CHAPTER 5. Dental hygienist.	
SECTION I. General	139
II. Structure and physiology	140-142
III. Dental caries	143-144
IV. Other diseases of mouth	145-153
V. Saliva, deposits, and accretions upon teeth	154-157

	Paragraphs
VI. Technique of dental prophylaxis	158–161
VII. System for instrumentation and polishing	162–165
VIII. Instructions to patient	166–167
IX. Preparations for mouth and teeth	168–170

CHAPTER 6. Dental assistant.

	Paragraphs
SECTION I. Requisites of dental assistant	171–172
II. Care of dental clinic	173–174
III. Sterilization of instruments and dressings	175–181
IV. Care of equipment and supplies	182–190
V. Duties at chair	191–200
VI. Daily routine in clinic	201

CHAPTER 7. Record clerk, dental service.

	Paragraphs
SECTION I. General duties and forms used	202–205
II. W. D., M. D. Form No. 57 (Report of Dental Service)	206–207
III. W. D., M. D. Form No. 79 (Register of Dental Patients)	208–210
IV. W. D., M. D. Form No. 18b (Statement of Expenditure of Special Dental Materials)	211–213
V. Daily work sheet	214
VI. Hospital clinic records	215–219
VII. W. D., A. G. O. forms	220–221
VIII. Dental survey	222–224
IX. Dental history of station	225–227

	Page
APPENDIX. List of references	191
INDEX	193

Chapter 1

GENERAL

                                                                                     Paragraph
Purpose and scope_____ 1

1. Purpose and scope.—*a.* Many complex problems confront the Dental Corps at the present time in the development of its various activities in the expansion program. One of the principal problems concerns the development of the laboratory service and the training of prosthetic technicians and enlisted personnel who are trained as dental assistants, record clerks, hygienists, and X-ray technicians. The entire training program depends very largely upon a standardization of the dental service. This also involves all the activities of enlisted personnel.

b. Chapters 3 to 7, inclusive, cover the essential phases and activities of the five assignments which, in the dental service, are usually filled by Medical Department enlisted men.

c. Chapter 2 is a general introduction to the technical aspects of the dental service and should be incorporated in the training program for all of the assigned dental personnel. The first sections of chapter 5 may be used as general information useful to all nonprofessional personnel with the dental service.

Chapter 2

MOUTH AND TEETH

	Paragraphs
Section I. General	2-3
II. Teeth	4-7
III. Regional anatomy	8-14
IV. Definitions	15

Section I

GENERAL

	Paragraph
Form and function	2
General structure	3

2. Form and function.—*a. Form.*—A dental technician should know something about the form and function of the mouth and teeth in order that he may have a complete knowledge of his work. As artificial restorations reproduce some or all of the teeth and some of the supporting structure, the dental technician must know the form of each tooth and its related parts in order that he may reproduce these teeth in the artificial substitute. This chapter deals with the mouth and teeth in a general way. It is very important that the dental technician have a detailed knowledge of the form and contour of each tooth so that he can carve reproductions of the teeth for artificial replacements. This study of the exact shape and contour of each tooth, known as dental anatomy, will be taken up in the study of tooth carving which will precede the technical work explained in this manual. This chapter is confined to a general study of the mouth and teeth, leaving the detailed tooth anatomy to be taken up with the exercises in tooth carving.

b. Function.—The mouth or oral cavity is man's organ for receiving food and for preparing that food for the first process of digestion, that is, dividing it into small parts by chewing and mixing it with the salivary secretions. Man's diet is both animal and vegetable (omnivorous). His teeth differ from the lower animals which are exclusively meat eaters (carnivorous) or vegetable eaters (herbivorous) and are formed for cutting, tearing, and grinding many kinds of foods. The incisor teeth situated in the front of the mouth have edges for cutting; the cuspids and bicuspids at the sides of the mouth have fairly sharp points or cusps for tearing; and the molars at the back part of the mouth have broad surfaces with low projections (cusps) for grinding the food.

DENTAL TECHNICIANS

3. General structure.—*a.* The mouth is bounded in back by the throat or pharynx and in front by the lips. Above, a vault separates the mouth cavity from the nasal passages. This vault is called the palate; and in the front and middle part it has a hard surface because it is composed of bone with a thin covering of gum tissue (mucous membrane) over it. This part is called the hard palate. Behind the bony portion a soft sheet of muscular tissue continues downward toward the throat and terminates in a small tonguelike projection, the uvula. This soft portion is called the soft palate (fig. 1). Sometimes

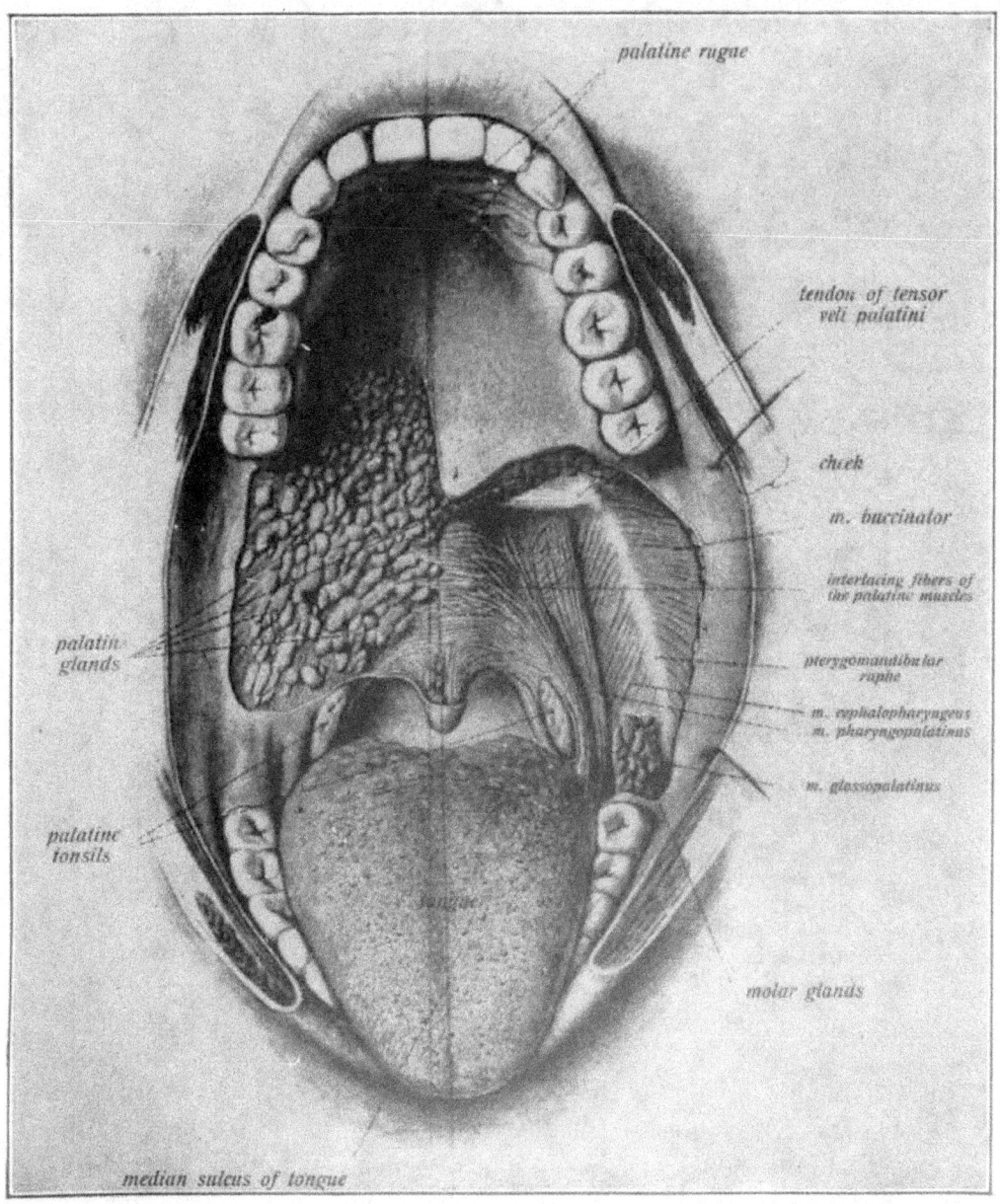

FIGURE 1.—Superior and posterior structures of oral cavity.

persons are born with a hole or aperture in the palate which allows a communication of the nose and mouth cavities. Such people are spoken of as having a cleft palate, and to provide for their speaking and eating normally, an operation must be performed to close this opening. Sometimes even after operation an opening into the nasal cavities persists, and an artificial plate must be made by the dentist for the patient to wear in his mouth to cover this aperture.

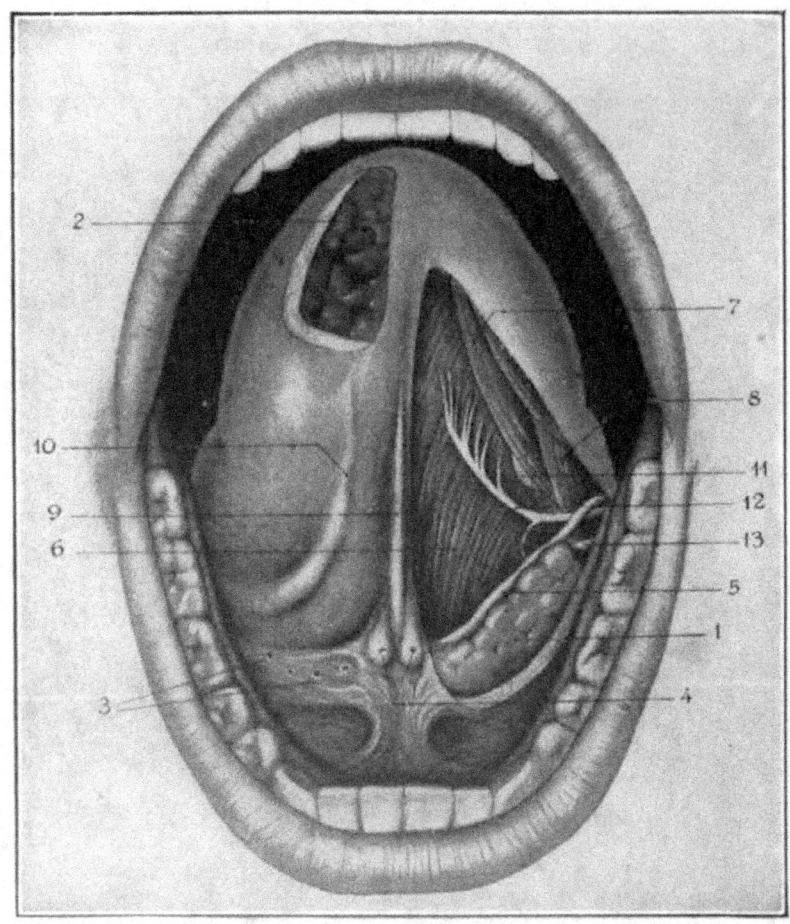

1. Sublingual gland.
2. Anterior gland of tongue.
3. Ducts of Rivinus.
4. Opening of submaxillary duct (Wharton's duct).
5. Submaxillary duct.
6. Genioglossus muscle.
7. Styloglossus muscle.
8. Hyoglossus muscle.
9. Frenum linguae.
10. Plica fimbriata.
11. Profunda lingual artery.
12. Lingual nerve.
13. Hypoglossal nerve.

FIGURE 2.—Structures of tongue and floor of mouth.

b. The floor of the mouth is a soft, thick, muscular layer which supports the front part of the tongue and in which are located some of the salivary glands (fig. 2). The tongue is attached to the upper part of the throat and to the floor of the mouth. It is a strong, muscular organ used in masticating food, in swallowing, and in talking. The teeth are firmly set in the jawbones. The upper jawbone is composed of two bones rigidly joined together, the right and left maxillary bones. These bones are also firmly attached to the other bones of the skull and face. The lower jaw is called the mandible. It is a strong, heavy, horseshoe-shaped bone attached to the skull on each side just in front of the ear canal by means of ball-and-socket type joints, the temporomandibular articulations. These joints permit a rather wide range of movement for opening the mouth and for chewing food.

Section II

TEETH

	Paragraph
Classification	4
Names and numbers	5
Surfaces	6
Roots	7

4. Classification.—*a.* Teeth are sometimes roughly divided into anterior and posterior. The anterior teeth are those toward the front of the mouth, and the posterior teeth are those toward the back of the mouth. The anterior teeth include the incisors and cuspids, while the posterior teeth include the bicuspids and molars.

b. Another general classification divides the teeth into incising and masticating; the incising teeth include the incisors and cuspids, and the masticating teeth include the bicuspids and molars.

5. Names and numbers.—*a.* There are 32 teeth in the human mouth; 16 in the upper jaw called the maxilla, and 16 in the lower jaw called the mandible. The teeth are called incisors, cuspids, bicuspids, and molars.

b. The median line is an imaginary perpendicular line drawn through the center of the body, dividing the body into right and left halves.

c. Taking the right side as an example, and starting at the median line, the teeth are named as follows:

Upper right central incisor.   Lower right central incisor.
Upper right lateral incisor.   Lower right lateral incisor.
Upper right cuspid.   Lower right cuspid.
Upper right first bicuspid.   Lower right first bicuspid.
Upper right second bicuspid.   Lower right second bicuspid.
Upper right first molar.   Lower right first molar.
Upper right second molar.   Lower right second molar.
Upper right third molar.   Lower right third molar.

The left side is the same, except that the word left is substituted for right.

d. Several systems of numbering the teeth have been devised whereby it is much simpler to designate a tooth by number rather than by name. The system in use in the Army is as follows:

(1) Beginning at the median line in the upper jaw and continuing backward, the teeth are numbered from 1 to 8; beginning at the median line in the lower jaw and continuing backward, the teeth are numbered from 9 to 16. Thus, a number between 1 and 8 would indicate that a tooth was an upper, whereas a number from 9 to 16 would indicate that the tooth was a lower. The letter R or L is placed in front of the number to designate whether the tooth is in the right or left side of the jaw.

(2) The following diagram may make this clearer:

Median line

Right								Left							
8	7	6	5	4	3	2	1	1	2	3	4	5	6	7	8
16	15	14	13	12	11	10	9	9	10	11	12	13	14	15	16

With this system when a tooth is designated as L3, it is known that the upper left cuspid is meant. R9 would be the lower right central incisor, R14 the lower right first molar, etc.

6. Surfaces.—Each tooth has five surfaces which can be compared roughly to the four sides and top of a box. Each side has a name to designate the various surfaces:

a. The mesial surface is the surface or side of the tooth nearest the median line.

b. The distal surface is the surface or side of the tooth farthest from the median line.

c. The buccal surface is the outside surface of the tooth or the side which lies next to the cheek. The term is usually applied to the bicuspids and molars.

d. The labial surface is the outside surface of the tooth or the side which lies next to the lips. The term is usually applied to the incisors and cuspids. The labial surface of the incisors and cuspids refers to the same side that is called the buccal surface in the case of the bicuspids and molars.

e. The facial surface is a term used to designate the side of the tooth next to the lips or cheeks and can be applied to either the anterior or posterior teeth. Labial, buccal, and facial all refer to the same surface of the teeth.

f. The lingual surface is the inner surface of the tooth or the side which lies next to the tongue.

g. The incisal surface or incisal edge is the cutting edge of the tooth and is used when speaking of this surface of the incisors and cuspids.

h. The occlusal surface is the top surface or grinding surface and is used when referring to this surface of the bicuspids and molars.

i. The entire name of the surface is ordinarily not used; instead, abbreviations which consist of the first letter of the word, as M, mesial, D, distal, O, occlusal, etc. Combinations of these letters are used to designate more than one surface. For instance, an inlay that extends over both the mesial and occlusal surfaces of a tooth is an MO inlay. Many combinations are used such as DO, LO, MI, MOD, etc.

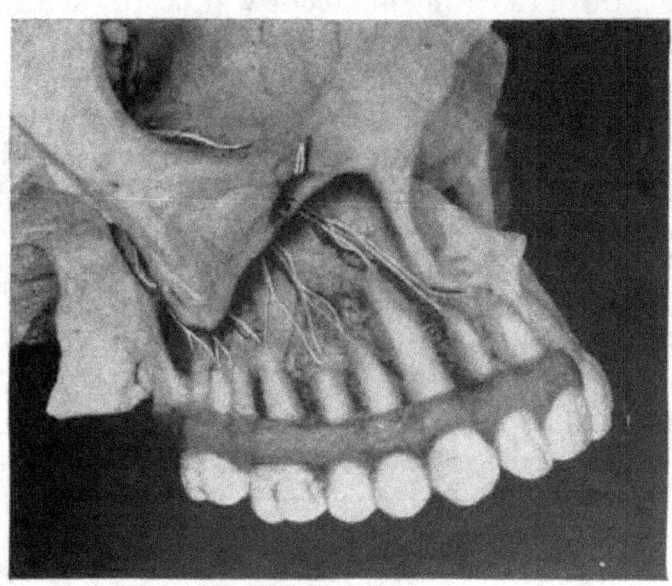

FIGURE 3.—Maxilla with outer plate of bone removed to show roots of teeth and their blood supply.

j. For descriptive purposes, the crown of a tooth is divided into thirds. The third nearest the incisal edge in the case of the incising teeth, or the occlusal surface in the case of the masticating teeth, is called the incisal third or occlusal third as the case may be. The next third is called the middle third, and the third next to the gum is called the gingival third.

7. Roots.—Dental technicians are not as much concerned with the roots of the teeth as with the crowns. However, a brief description of them is given below.

a. The central incisors, lateral incisors, and cuspids, in both the upper and lower jaws, are all single-rooted teeth. The upper cuspids have the longest and heaviest roots of any of the teeth. The lower central incisors have the shortest and smallest roots.

b. The upper first bicuspid usually has two frail roots, one placed buccally and the other lingually. It is not uncommon for the two roots to be fused together, giving the appearance of one single root. The upper second bicuspids are nearly always single rooted.

c. The upper first molar has three roots, two on the buccal and one on the lingual.

d. The upper second molar generally has three roots and is quite similar to the first molar except that there is more tendency for the roots to be fused together.

e. The upper third molar may have from one to five roots or even more. Often, three roots in this tooth will be fused together so as to form one big cone-shaped root. At other times there will be three or four small frail roots. The upper third molar and lower third molar are subject to far greater variation than any of the other teeth. Figure 3 shows the roots of the upper teeth, the bone being cut away to demonstrate position of the roots.

f. The lower bicuspids, both first and second, are single-rooted.

g. The lower first molar has two roots, one mesial and one distal.

h. The lower second molar is similar to the first, except that there is more tendency for the roots to fuse together.

i. The lower third molar, like the upper third molar, is subject to great variation. Two roots are probably as commonly found as any other number, although very often there is only one, or there may be three or four.

Section III

REGIONAL ANATOMY

	Paragraph
Relation to dental prosthesis	8
Hard and soft palates	9
Mandible	10
Temporomandibular articulation	11
Muscles of mastication	12
Frena of mouth	13
Torus palatinus	14

8. Relation to dental prosthesis.—Section I referred to the parts of the mouth other than the teeth: the hard and soft palate, lips and cheeks, tongue, uvula, and maxillary bones and joints. A dental technician could do his work very well without a knowledge of these parts but he will have a better understanding of his work if he knows something of the anatomy of the mouth. In full denture work, especially, many steps are taken to conform the denture to the struc- the mouth. There are certain areas over which excessive pressure is undesirable, and the denture must be scraped or relieved in these areas during its construction. The subject of anatomy with its peculiar names is a difficult one at best. However, the following is simplified as much as possible and should be accompanied by demonstrations by the instructors on models and skulls which will make it easier to understand.

9. **Hard and soft palates.**—*a.* The hard palate is the roof of the mouth. It is formed by the union of the horizontal portions of the maxillary bones and palate bones at the median line. The front and side borders of the hard palate consist of that portion of the bone which gives support to the teeth. The posterior border is irregular and has attached to it a muscularlike curtain which is called the soft palate. The hard palate is covered throughout by a thick, firm, mucous membrane which is closely adherent to the bone.

b. In the center of the hard palate is a prominent bony ridge covered by mucous membrane. This ridge is called the *palatal raphe* or *median raphe* and indicates the line of union formed during the development of the parts. Near the center of the hard palate the raphe frequently separates into two smaller ridges which continue backward, side by side, thus making it appear wider here than toward the front or back. As it runs posteriorly the raphe usually diminishes in size, disappearing entirely as the soft palate is approached, although occasionally it is quite pronounced the entire length of the hard palate.

c. This ridge is usually much harder and less compressible than the mucous membrane on either side of it. Unless one relieves the denture over this hard area and allows it to rest evenly over the entire surface of the roof of the mouth, the denture will rock in the mouth, using the raphe as a fulcrum. This condition not only causes the denture to be unsatisfactory as to fit, but also causes a soreness over the ridge. A continued irritation of this kind over a period of time might even be the cause of a malignant growth.

d. On either side of this central ridge, or raphe, in the anterior part of the mouth are found a number of fantastically arranged folds of mucous membrane which are called rugae. The number and size of these folds vary considerably. In some cases they are quite numerous and very prominent, while in other cases they are few in number and only slightly developed.

e. At the anterior end of the raphe and just behind the central incisors there is an opening in the bone which is called the anterior palatal foramen through which certain nerves and blood vessels pass.

f. At the back part of the hard palate are two other openings in the bone which are called the posterior palatal foramina. These are found on either side of the hard palate and are located about halfway between the median line and the gingival border of the molars, and about 5 millimeters anterior to the junction of the hard and soft palate.

g. These openings and their positions are important because it is often necessary to relieve over these areas on dentures. Nerves and blood vessels pass through them, and in some cases excessive pressure by the denture over these areas will cause a very uncomfortable burning sensation over the roof of the patient's mouth unless proper relief has been made. Figure 4 shows the tissues taken off to expose these foramina and demonstrates, on the left side of the figure, the blood vessels and nerves.

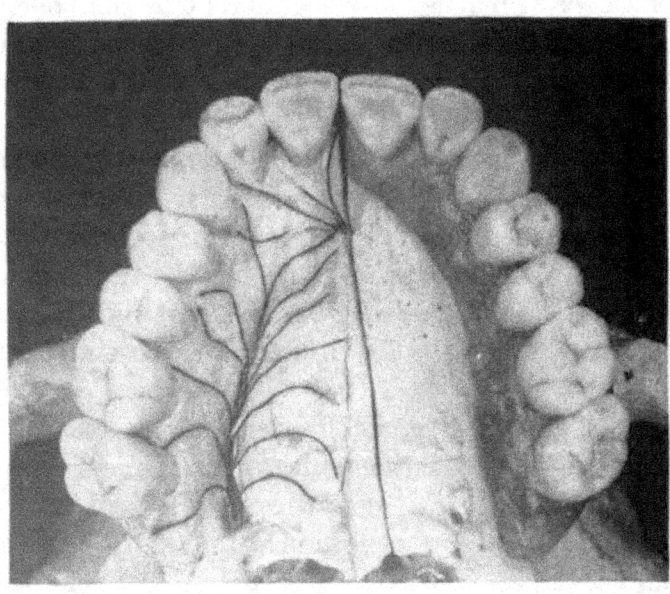

FIGURE 4.—Hard palate showing foramina and (on left side) blood vessels and nerves which emerge from them.

h. The soft palate is attached to the posterior border of the hard palate from which it is continued as a backward prolongation of its soft tissue. It runs downward and backward, and forms part of the posterior border of the oral cavity. The soft palate is composed of thin, dense, muscular fibers, blood vessels, nerves, and mucous glands. It has no underlying bony support. In short, the hard palate is the part of the roof of the mouth with underlying bony support, whereas the soft palate is the part with no bony support. The soft palate is movable, but the hard palate is not. The posterior border of a denture should never end on the hard palate; it should always extend a distance onto the soft palate.

10. Mandible.—*a.* The mandible or lower jawbone is the heaviest and strongest bone of the head. It supports the 16 lower teeth and serves as a framework for the floor of the mouth. It is movable, having no bony union with the skull proper. It is attached to the skull by movable joints called the temporomandibular articulations, which will be taken up in detail later on. The mandible is symmetrical in form and consists of a horizontal portion called the body, and two vertical portions each of which is called a ramus (fig. 5).

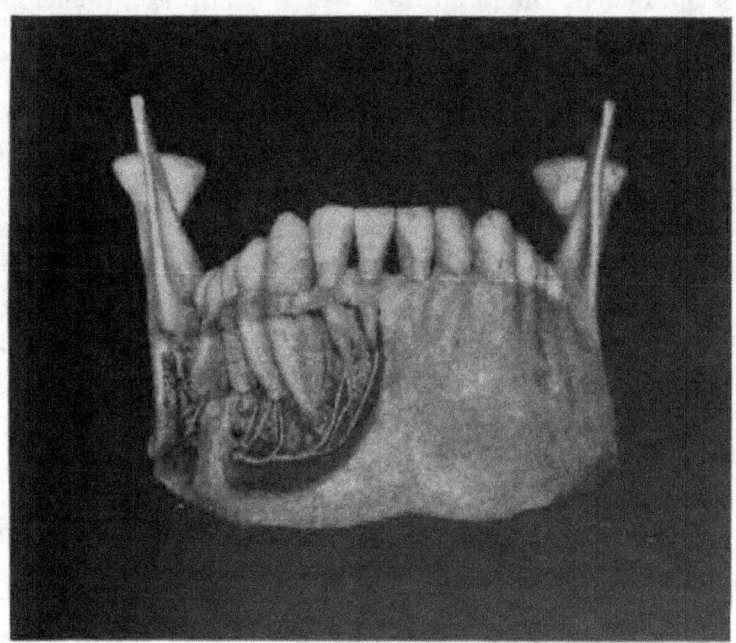

FIGURE 5.—Anterior view of mandible with outer plate of bone removed on left side of figure to demonstrate roots of teeth and blood and nerve supply.

b. The mandible forms from two centers and consists of two identical halves which meet at the median line forming a slight vertical ridge which indicates the line of union of the two halves. This ridge or junction is called the symphysis. Each half of the mandible has two surfaces, an inner and an outer one, and on each surface are certain points or landmarks which should be recognized.

c. The external oblique line is a well-defined ridge extending obliquely across the facial or outer surface of the mandible. It extends from the mental process upward and backward to the base of the vertical portion of the bone, and is continuous with the anterior border of the vertical portion or ramus.

d. The mental foramen is an opening in the bone usually situated about halfway between the upper and lower borders of the body of the mandible, and between the roots of the first and second bicuspid teeth. It gives passage to certain nerves and accompanying b' vessels. Ordinarily, because of its position, no pressure is exerted on this nerve by a denture, and no relief is necessary. However, in very old persons where teeth have been absent a long time, the bone has absorbed a great deal, and the foramen is found very close to the upper border of the body of the mandible. In these cases it sometimes becomes necessary to relieve the denture over this area to avoid excessive pressure with resulting pain.

e. The mylohyoid ridge or internal oblique ridge is a heavy ridge on the inner surface of the mandible, which occupies a position closely corresponding to the external oblique line on the facial surface. It begins near the base of the bone at the median line, and passes backward and upward, increasing in prominence until the base of the vertical portion of the bone is reached, into which it gradually disappears.

f. The inferior dental foramen or mandibular foramen is an opening in the bone located near the center of the inner surface of the ramus of the mandible. It is the entrance to the mandibular canal which passes downward and forward through the ramus and body of the mandible finding an exit at the mental foramen on the external surface of the mandible.

g. The mylohyoid groove is a depression or groove found on the inner surface of the mandible. It starts at the base of the mandibular foramen and runs obliquely downward and forward below the mylohyoid or internal oblique ridge. It accommodates the nerves and blood vessels which supply the floor of the mouth.

h. The sigmoid notch is the crescent-shaped upper border of the ramus of the mandible.

i. The anterior portion of the notch is formed by a flattened cone-shaped projection called the coronoid process which serves as an attachment for one of the muscles of mastication.

j. The posterior portion of the notch is formed by a rounded or oblong projection which is called the condyloid process. The condyloid process, or condyle, is the portion of the mandible that enters into the formation of the joint which is referred to as the temporomandibular articulation. The condyle is divided into two sections: a head which is the rounded upper portion of the process and neck which is the somewhat constricted portion joining the head to the main body of the ramus.

11. Temporomandibular articulation.—*a.* Attention has already been called to the fact that the mandible has no bony union with the skull proper, but is attached to it by a movable joint. It is this joint or attachment that is known as the temporomandibular articulation. It receives its name from the two bones which enter into its formation, the temporal bone and the mandible.

b. This joint is the seat of motion in the mandible, and entering into its construction are bones, ligaments, cartilage, and synovial membrane. These are the tissues essential to all movable articulations. The various movable joints of the body are classified according to the nature of the movement; and they correspond to the mechanical actions known as hinge joint, ball and socket joint, gliding joint, pulley joint, etc. The temporomandibular joint is a combination of the gliding type and hinge type.

c. The bony parts entering into the formation of this joint are the glenoid fossa of the temporal bone and condyloid process of the mandible. The glenoid fossa is a rounded cavity or depression, in the temporal bone, into which the head of the condyle fits to form the joint.

d. The movement of the jaw is not limited to a simple opening and closing motion. The jaw is protruded (pushed forward), or retruded (pushed backward). There are also lateral movements in which the mandible is moved to either side. All of these various movements and the function of the teeth are closely associated with the temporomandibular articulation, and for this reason it is important to understand how it is constructed. The articulators used are made so that more or less normal movements of the mandible can be reproduced, the metal parts which form the joint of the articulator being similar to the bony parts forming the temporomandibular articulation.

e. There is a wide variation in this joint in various individuals, and in many cases the same person will have considerable variation between the joint on his right side and that on his left side.

f. In nonadjustable articulators an average joint has been built into the articulator which fits most cases fairly well. Cases which vary greatly from the average, or cases in which there is considerable difference in the right and left temporomandibular articulations, will not be as satisfactory when built on the nonadjustable type of articulator as when they are constructed on an adjustable type.

g. Adjustable articulators are so constructed that the angles of the joints of the articulator can be varied and set to reproduce exactly the angles of the temporomandibular articulation of the patient. Group demonstrations will be given in which the temporomandibular articulation in a skull will be compared with the temporomandibular articulation as it is reproduced in the articulator.

12. Muscles of mastication.—Occupying the back part of the side of the face and forming an independent group are four muscles which are usually classed as the muscles of mastication. While this is true to a great degree, they are not the only muscles brought into action during this process. These four muscles of mastication are—

>   Masseter.
>   Temporal.
>   Internal pterygoid.
>   External pterygoid.

Each one will be taken up separately. As stated previously, some difficulty will be experienced with the anatomical terms used. However, in the group demonstrations everything will be pointed out on a skull to demonstrate where the muscles are attached and what their general action is, even though the origin and insertion of each muscle by its proper name may not be known. Generally speaking. the masseter, temporal, and internal pterygoid elevate or close the lower jaw, the principal function of the external pterygoid being to extend the lower jaw so that the lower teeth pass beyond the upper. The muscles which depress the jaw are certain muscles of the neck which will not be considered.

a. Masseter.—This muscle extends generally from the zygomatic arch and the lower border of the malar bone, downward and backward to the outer surface of the ramus of the mandible. It is a strong, heavy muscle whose main action is to draw the jaw slightly forward and to close the jaw.

b. Temporal.—This is a large fan-shaped muscle whose broad end is attached to the entire surface of the temporal fossa. From here it extends downward passing underneath the zygomatic arch, and is attached at its narrow end to the coronoid process of the mandible. Its action is to close the lower jaw, some of its fibers drawing the jaw backward after certain other muscles have protruded it.

c. Internal pterygoid.—The internal pterygoid is attached at one end to the inner surface of the external pterygoid plate, the tuberosity of the palate bone, and a small portion of the maxilla. From here it extends downward, backward, and outward, its other end being attached to the internal surface of the ramus of the mandible at its lower and posterior borders. It is a thick, sheetlike muscle whose action is to close the jaw; at the same time the action draws the jaw backward and throws it toward the opposite side.

d. External pterygoid.—The external pterygoid is composed of t heads, an upper and a lower. The upper head arises from the greater wing of the sphenoid bone and from the internal pterygoid ridge. It is inserted into the interarticular cartilage, into the capsule of the joint, and into the neck of the condyle. The lower head arises from the outer surface of the external pterygoid plate and is inserted into the neck of the condyle. The action of this muscle is to draw the condyle and interarticular cartilage forward and inward. The combination of these two movements produces an oblique movement of the lower molars with respect to the opposing upper molars.

13. **Frena of mouth.**—In various situations about the labial, buccal, and lingual surfaces of the gums, small slender folds of mucous membrane are found extending into the surrounding tissues. These folds, which act as a bridle or curb to the adjacent movable parts, are known as the frena of the mouth. The principal frena, three in number, are found at the median line and are named as follows:

>Frenum labium superioris.
>Frenum labium inferioris.
>Frenum linguae.

a. The frenum labium superioris extends from the inner surface of the upper lip to the upper gum, and limits to some extent the movement of the upper lip. Its attachment to the gum is quite variable, sometimes being attached very high, and in other cases extending down to the gingival border of the teeth. The frenum labium superioris is usually much larger than the frenum labium inferioris.

b. The frenum labium inferioris extends from the inner surface of the lower lip to the lower gum, and limits to some extent the movement of the lower lip. As in the upper, the attachment to the gum is variable. This frenum is the smallest of the three principal frena and in some cases is so small that it cannot be seen unless the lip is stretched.

c. The frenum linguae extends from the under surface of the tip of the tongue to the lingual surface of the lower gums at the median line. This frenum limits the movement of the tongue to some extent and is the largest and strongest of the three principal frena. It is much stronger than those connected with the lips.

d. Similar bridles are found in the buccal region, usually near the bicuspid teeth, but they are much smaller than those at the median line. The frena are of great importance because allowance must be made for them in constructing dentures. If a denture i̇ structed without the proper allowance having been made for the frena, it will be a matter of only a few hours until they are so sore that the denture cannot be worn.

14. Torus palatinus.—This is a condition occasionally confronted with in making dentures. It consists of a bony protuberance covered with mucous membrane. It is usually found in the roof of the mouth. The protuberance varies greatly in size in different individuals. Some are quite small, while others are so large that they almost fill the vault of the mouth. In most cases they should probably be removed surgically, but for one reason or another they are frequently not removed, and it is necessary to construct dentures over them. They are hard, like the median raphe, and good relief must always be made over them for the same reasons as for the median raphe. These reasons are to permit a more perfect fit by eliminating rocking of the denture, and to avoid soreness over these areas and eliminate the possibility of malignant growths developing due to long-continued irritation. This condition is occasionally found in other locations about the mouth. Probably the next most common place is on the lingual surface of the mandible in the region of the cuspids and bicuspids.

SECTION IV

DEFINITIONS

Paragraph
Terms used_____ 15

15. Terms used.—*a.* Without considerable previous training, many terms will be found confusing or meaningless, but they must be known because they will be encountered as long as there is any connection with dentistry. Definitions of the more important of these follow:

Alloy.—A metal composed of two or more different metals which have been mixed in the molten state. In dentistry alloys used are generally a mixture of gold and one or more other metals such as copper, silver, etc. These metallic mixtures are called gold alloys.

Alveolar process.—The projection of the maxillary bones which envelops the roots of the teeth and forms their alveoli (sockets).

Alveolus.—The cavity or socket in the bone in which the root of a tooth is embedded or fixed

Apex.—The terminal end of the root of a tooth.

Axial surfaces.—Those surfaces of the teeth that are parallel with their long axes. They are labial, buccal, linqual, mesial, and distal.

Bell-crowned.—A tooth in which the mesio-distal diameter of the crown is much greater than that of the neck.

Cementum.—A tissue resembling bone which forms the outer surface of the roots of the teeth.

Contact point.—The point on the proximal surface of a tooth which touches a neighboring tooth.

Crown.—That portion of a tooth which is covered with enamel and which projects from the tissues in which the root is fixed

Cusp.—A pronounced elevation or point on the surface of a tooth, more especially on the occlusal surface.

Cutting edge.—The edge formed by the junction of the labial and lingual surfaces of the incisor and cuspid teeth. In the cuspids the edge is raised to a point near its center.

Deciduous teeth.—The teeth of the child which are shed to give place to the permanent teeth. They are sometimes referred to as temporary teeth, baby teeth, milk teeth, etc.

Dentine.—The hard tissue of which the main body of a tooth is formed.

Embrasure.—An opening that widens outward or inward. That portion of the interproximal space that widens toward the buccal or toward the lingual.

Enamel.—A very hard tissue covering the crown of a tooth.

Facial.—The outside surface of a tooth which is adjacent to the face.

Fissure.—A *fault* in the surface of a tooth caused by the imperfect joining of the enamel of the different lobes. Fissures occur along the lines of the developmental grooves.

Foramen (pl. *foramina*).—An opening in the surface of a bone (or at the apex of a tooth) for the passage of blood vessels and nerve fibers.

Fossa.—A round or angular depression in the surface of a tooth. These occur mostly in the occlusal surfaces of the molars and in the lingual surfaces of the incisors.

Gingiva.—The portion of gum tissue enveloping the necks of the teeth crownwise from the attachment at the gingival line. A shorter definition is the free margin of the gum.

Gingival line.—The line around the neck of a tooth at which the gingiva is attached. The line of junction of the enamel and cementum.

Groove.—A long-shaped depression in the surface of a tooth.

Inclination.—The inclination of a tooth is the deviation of the long axis of the tooth from the perpendicular.

Interproximal embrasure.—That portion of the interproximal space which widens toward the lip or cheek, or toward the tor

Interproximal space.—The V-shaped space between adjoining teeth. This space is formed by the proximal surfaces of the adjoining teeth and the border of the alveolar process between the necks of the teeth. Normally this space is filled with gum tissue.

Marginal ridge.—The ridges, or elevations, of enamel on the margins of the occlusal surfaces of the bicuspids and molars and on the mesial and distal margins of the lingual surfaces of the incisors and cuspids.

Median line.—An imaginary perpendicular line drawn through the center of the body, which divides the body into right and left halves.

Neck.—That portion of the tooth which forms the junction of the crown and root.

Oblique ridge.—A ridge running obliquely across the occlusal surface of the upper molars. It is formed by the union of the triangular ridge of the disto-buccal cusp with the distal portion of the ridge forming the mesio-lingual cusp.

Pit.—A sharp pointed depression in the enamel. Pits occur mostly where several developmental grooves join, as in the occlusal surfaces of the molars, and at the endings of the buccal grooves on the buccal surfaces of the molars.

Proximal surface.—The surface of a tooth which lies next to another tooth. This nearly always means mesial or distal.

Ridge.—A long-shaped elevation on the surface of a tooth.

Rugae.—A series of irregular ridges on the front part of the roof of the mouth.

Septum.—That portion of the alveolar process which lies between the roots of the teeth separating their alveoli.

Sulcus.—A notable long-shaped depression in the surface of a tooth, the inclines of which meet at an angle. A sulcus has a developmental groove at the junction of its inclines.

Supplemental groove.—A shallow long-shaped depression in the surface of a tooth, generally with a smoothly rounded bottom. Supplemental grooves differ from development grooves in that they do not mark the junction of lobes.

Supplemental lobe.—A lobe that does not belong to the typical form of the tooth; an additional lobe.

Supplemental ridge.—A ridge on the surface of a tooth that does not belong to the typical form of the tooth; an additional ridge.

Transverse ridge.—A ridge formed of two triangular ridges, which join to form a continuous ridge across the occlusal surface of a tooth.

Triangular ridge.—A ridge running from the point of a cusp toward the central portion of the occlusal surface of a tooth.

Tubercle.—A slight rounded elevation on the surface of a tooth. Tubercles occur frequently on the linguo-gingival ridge of the incisors and occasionally upon various parts of other teeth. They are deviations from typical tooth forms.

b. See appendix for list of references.

Chapter 3

PROSTHETIC TECHNICIAN

	Paragraphs
Section I. General	16
II. Impression materials	17
III. Plaster impressions	18–22
IV. Modeling compound impressions	23–25
V. Hydrocolloid impressions	26
VI. Construction of full and partial vulcanite dentures	27–48
VII. Acrylic resin dentures	49–50
VIII. Denture repair	51–58
IX. Dental castings	59–62
X. Cast crowns	63–65
XI. Cast occlusal gold crown	66–67
XII. Fixed bridge	68–71
XIII. Clasps and bars for partial dentures	72–78
XIV. Cast partial dentures and partial denture skeletons	79–93
XV. Splints	94–97

Section I

GENERAL

	Paragraph
Scope	16

16. Scope.—The term prosthetic dentistry or prosthodontia may be defined as that branch of dentistry which has to do with the replacement of any lost or missing parts of the dental apparatus by suitable artificial substitutes. Dental laboratory mechanics is that part of the science or art of prosthodontia which has to do with the construction of these appliances. The instructions contained in this chapter include the laboratory procedures for the construction of full dentures, partial dentures, crowns, bridges, and splints. A full denture may be defined as a structure replacing the full number of teeth in either jaw. A partial denture is a structure replacing the missing natural teeth in either jaw and is retained by mechanical means against the remaining natural teeth. A crown is an artificial restoration of the crown of a natural tooth. A bridge is a fixed appliance which replaces lost teeth, retained by attachments other than clasps to abutments supported by the roots or crowns of adjoining teeth. A splint is any apparatus, appliance, or device employed to prevent motion or displacement of fractured or movable parts.

DENTAL TECHNICIANS

Section II

IMPRESSION MATERIALS

	Paragraph
Description and limitations	17

17. Description and limitations.—An impression is an exact negative reproduction of a patient's oral arch and teeth. A positive form or cast is obtained from the impression that is identical to the mouth. The dental technician's work begins when he receives the completed impression from the dental officer. As a great deal of painstaking care is needed to secure an accurate impression, the importance of skillful handling of the impression by the technician cannot be stressed too much. Any deviation from this will result in the completed denture being unsatisfactory. In an edentulous or toothless mouth there are usually no undercuts present, or at least very few. Therefore no great problem is presented in getting the impression from the mouth. For this reason a material such as modeling compound can be used. This material becomes plastic upon the addition of heat and returns to its hard state when allowed to cool in the mouth. However, a dental arch containing some natural teeth presents quite a different problem; that is, one concerning the selection of a suitable impression material. As can be seen by looking in any mouth, there are always undercuts when natural teeth are present. If an impression of this type was taken in modeling compound, it would be very difficult to remove and when once removed, it would be distorted to such an extent as to render it useless. Therefore another type of impression material must be used. There are two materials commonly used for this type of case, each having entirely different characteristics, but both giving equally good results. The first is plaster of paris, which is placed in the mouth while in its plastic stage and allowed to set. It is then broken into several fragments, which permits its removal from the mouth, and at the same time preserves the details of all the undercuts. These fragments are later reassembled in their proper relationship, which gives an accurate reproduction of the dental arch. The other type of impression material is the hydrocolloid. This material can be softened by moist heat, placed in the mouth, and allowed to cool. Due to its great elasticity, it can be removed over the undercuts without any distortion of the impression. Various combinations of materials may also be used, and these will be discussed later.

Section III

PLASTER IMPRESSIONS

	Paragraph
General	18
Assembling parts	19
Boxing	20
Pouring casts	21
Separating casts	22

18. General.—Plaster impressions for partial dentures consist of several pieces that must be reassembled in the tray in their proper position and relationship. Great care must be taken in the handling of these broken fragments, as any further breakage or rubbing of the edges will seriously interfere with the accuracy of the impression. The steps taken in the assembling of the plaster impression are as given in paragraph 19.

19. Assembling parts.—*a.* Allow the fragments to dry before beginning to assemble the impression.

b. Remove all crumbs of plaster from the tray.

c. Gently remove all adhering particles of plaster from the fractured edges of the impression with a camel's-hair brush.

d. Assemble the parts in the tray consecutively so as to avoid undercuts. Never force any fragment in position, as this will mar the edges. If the pieces are assembled in the proper order, they will easily slip into their correct places.

e. After the parts are assembled in the tray, apply a slight amount of finger pressure on the various pieces of plaster so that the lines of fracture are barely noticeable. Be sure that the entire impression fits snugly in the tray.

f. Maintain this pressure, and with a warm spatula carefully apply sticky wax to join the edges of the impression to the tray. Never allow the wax to touch the tissue surfaces of the impression.

g. With a camel's-hair brush, apply an alcoholic solution of orange shellac to the impression. It must be thin enough to penetrate the plaster to a slight degree without obliterating any of the fine details. This is used as a staining medium. Allow to dry.

h. With a camel's-hair brush, apply a coat of sandarac varnish over the shellacked surface of the impression and allow to dry. It should be thin enough so as not to obliterate the fine details. The varnish may be made thinner with a little alcohol, if necessary. This is used as a separating medium and the impression should now have a glossy, smooth finish. A solution of soap in water may be used in place of sandarac varnish as a separating medium.

20. Boxing.—The impression is now ready to be "boxed" preparatory to the pouring of the model. By this step the impression is reenforced by a retaining wall which confines the stone to the impression and simplifies the trimming of the cast after it is poured.

a. With a sharp knife, cut a strip about 3/16 inch in width along the entire length of the strip of boxing wax.

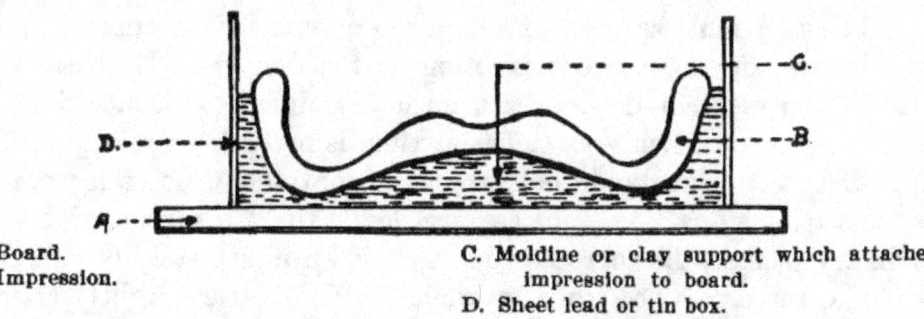

A. Board.
B. Impression.
C. Moldine or clay support which attaches impression to board.
D. Sheet lead or tin box.

FIGURE 6.—Boxing of upper impression by method not requiring heat.

b. Seal this strip around the outer edges of the impression about 1/8 inch away from the crest of the impression's rim and across the posterior border. Care should be exercised to prevent the wax from covering any portion of the impression.

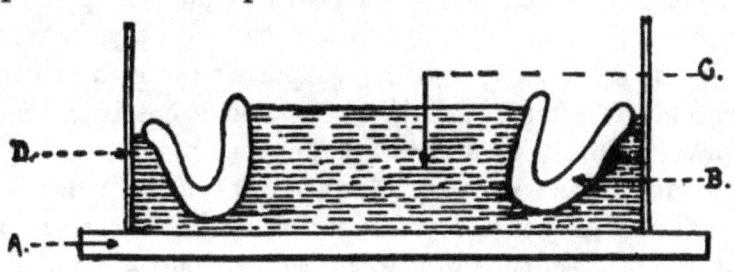

A. Board.
B. Impression.
C. Clay, moldine, or plaster support.
D. Sheet lead or tin box.

FIGURE 7.—Boxing of lower impression.

c. Mold the balance of the boxing wax to the outer border of the impression. With a warm spatula, seal the wax to the impression and along the edges of the boxing wax itself. Before sealing it is necessary to make certain that the top of the wax is not too high from the top of the impression, as this will create needless bulk in the cast; 1/3 inch is sufficient (fig. 6).

d. The technique for lower impressions is exactly the same, with the exception of one step. In the lower it is necessary to apply a small piece of moldine or wax in the space that is occupied by the tongue. After this has been done, the case is boxed as described above

21. Pouring casts.—This consists of transforming a negative impression of the dental arch into a positive reproduction of the same arch.

　a. After the plaster impression has been shellacked, varnished, and boxed, it should be immersed in water for 10 minutes prior to pouring the cast. This is to allow the plaster to absorb a certain amount of water which will make the later separation much easier, and also will prevent a chalky cast.

　b. Remove impression from water and dry off all excess moisture.

　c. The casts must be made of a material of sufficient strength to withstand usage during the construction of the denture. It must withstand the pressure and temperature changes during vulcanization. It must not set too quickly as sufficient time is needed for manipulation, and when setting it should not expand or contract. Such a material is quick-setting stone. As stone requires less water for mixing than does ordinary plaster, the correct proportion is approximately one part of water to three parts of stone by weight. This varies slightly according to the manufacturer, and his directions should be followed.

　d. Place the correct proportions of stone and water in a clean plaster bowl. Tap the bowl gently against the bench so that all air bubbles will be expelled. Leave sufficient time for the stone to absorb the water as this will aid in the spatulation.

　e. Hold the bowl in one hand, and with a plaster spatula mix the stone with a cutting motion until it assumes a puttylike consistency. Never whip the stone as this will incorporate air into the mix. Excessive spatulation after a puttylike consistency has been secured will reduce working time, a condition which must be guarded against.

　f. Never add water to a mix after spatulation in order to make it thinner. If such is done, crystallization which already has begun will be broken up resulting in a weak cast. Place a small portion of this stone in the rear of the impression, which is held in the hand. Gently jar it against the bench until the mix covers the tissue surface of the impression with a thin layer of stone.

　g. Continue adding the stone and allow each addition to settle in the impression before the next is deposited. Continue adding the stone until the impression is completely filled. Wait until the mix sets before proceeding.

　h. Remove boxing wax and score the top of the cast with a sharp knife to facilitate attachment to plaster when mounting on the articulator.

22. Separating casts.—*a.* With a sharp knife very carefully scrape off the impression plaster until the brown color of the staining material becomes visible. This will weaken the impression so that it will be easy to remove without injuring the cast.

b. Insert the sharp point of a knife in the line of fracture and apply slight pressure away from the teeth and thin parts of the cast. It is best to remove the plaster from around the teeth and undercuts before removing that from around the tissue surfaces. Great care must be taken in this step to prevent the breaking of teeth on the model.

c. Remove any adhering separating media from the casts with cotton and alcohol.

d. All rough edges and overhanging margins are removed with knife, file, or sandpaper, and the casts trimmed and shaped as desired.

Section IV

MODELING COMPOUND IMPRESSIONS

	Paragraph
General	23
Boxing	24
Separating cast	25

23. General.—A large percentage of the impressions that a dental technician must work with is taken in impression compound. It may be white, black, red, or brown in color. The boxing of the compound impression will require more care than those made from plaster. Whereas plaster that has hardened or set is unaffected by the application of hot wax in the boxing process, the compound will absorb some of the latent heat from the wax and soften sufficiently to distort it under hand manipulation, thus ruining the impression. Therefore it must be boxed by a method that does not require heat. A simple technique is given in paragraph 24.

24. Boxing.—*a.* Place the impression on some moldine or art clay which is molded to give evenly distributed support to the impression. This material is carried around the labial and buccal flanges of the impression to within $\frac{1}{8}$ inch from the crest of the impression and its posterior border. The sides should be perpendicular. A piece of tin or lead sheet is conformed to the periphery of the impression and held secure by elastic bands. The casts may then be poured without danger of distortion (fig. 6).

b. The method of handling the mandibular or lower impression is similar but the tongue area space of the lower requires a different treatment. The impression is seated on some moldine or art clay which is carried around the outside flanges as in the maxillary impression. Then the clay or moldine is carried into the tongue area space, filling it up to within ⅛ inch from the crest of the lingual flanges. A strip of tin or lead sheet is then carried around the circumference of the impression as before, and held with elastic bands. The cast is then poured. If it is impossible to obtain the moldine used in this technique, ordinary plaster may be used in its place. It is a little harder to manipulate but will serve the same purpose (fig. 7).

c. The modeling compound impressions do not need a staining and separating media unless a plaster wash has been used. This consists of a compound impression with a very thin layer of plaster over the entire tissue surface. In an impression of this type it is necessary to apply a light coat of sandarac varnish to the surface of the plaster so that the casts may be more readily separated from the impression. A staining coat of shellac is unnecessary.

25. Separating cast.—*a.* In the removal of the compound impression from the cast, it is necessary to apply sufficient heat to return the compound to a soft or plastic state. This is accomplished by immersing the impression in warm water for a sufficient length of time to allow the entire thickness of the compound to become soft. If the water is too hot, the compound will become sticky and will adhere to the cast.

b. Insert a knife blade under the edge of the impression and gently ease the compound away from the model. If it is sufficiently plastic, it should come away very easily. If it is too hard, there is danger of breaking the model. Take a small section at a time and then return the impression to the warm water for additional heating. In this way gradually remove the entire impression from the cast.

c. The cast is then trimmed and shaped as usual.

SECTION V

HYDROCOLLOID IMPRESSIONS

Paragraph
General _____ 26

26. General.—The third type of impression material that is commonly used is the hydrocolloid. It possesses unusual plasticity, some elasticity, and slight compressibility. The impression can be removed from undercuts without distortion and gives the finest detail. Casts are obtained without the use of separating media and without the danger of injury or breakage incident to the removal of the impression compound. Duplicate casts may be obtained by the careful removal of the model from the impression and repouring the impression or by making a second impression of the cast. This material is generally used in the making of impressions for partial dentures, although it may be used in conjunction with modeling compound for full denture cases. In either case, it is treated the same by the dental technician. The cast must be poured immediately after the impression is taken, otherwise the material will dry out and distort the impression. If this is impossible, it may be kept in cold water for a short time and then poured.

Section VI

CONSTRUCTION OF FULL AND PARTIAL VULCANITE DENTURES

	Paragraph
Relief areas	27
Trial denture base	28
Biteplates	29
Mounting casts on articulator	30
Selecting artificial teeth	31
Requirements of tooth forms	32
Arranging upper anteriors	33
Arranging upper posteriors	34
Arranging lower first molar	35
Arranging lower second bicuspid	36
Arranging lower anteriors	37
Arranging cuspids	38
Arranging lower first bicuspid	39
Incising bite	40
Balancing bite	41
Central dental laboratory assortment of new Trubyte teeth	42
Denture waxing	43
Denture flasking (full)	44
Denture flasking (partial)	45
Packing the case	46
Vulcanizing	47
Cleansing and polishing dentures	48

27. Relief areas.—The mucous membrane covering the bony tissues of the mouth is not of uniform thickness over the entire surface. There are areas where the membrane is very thin and the bone is quite prominent. This is especially true along the median raphe of the palate and the crest of the ridge. There are other areas of the mouth that have an abundance of connective tissue overlying the bone, examples of which are the tissue-bearing areas of the palate and the slopes of the ridge. In constructing a denture it is necessary to relieve these hard areas so that the soft tissues overlying them will not be compressed when the denture is worn, and at the same time allow the tissue-bearing areas to be evenly compressed. In addition to these bony areas, it is sometimes necessary to relieve pressure on nerves and blood vessels, especially where they come through the bony openings. Relief areas may be prepared in two ways:

　a. The dental officer may prepare the areas to be relieved in the impression before the cast is made.

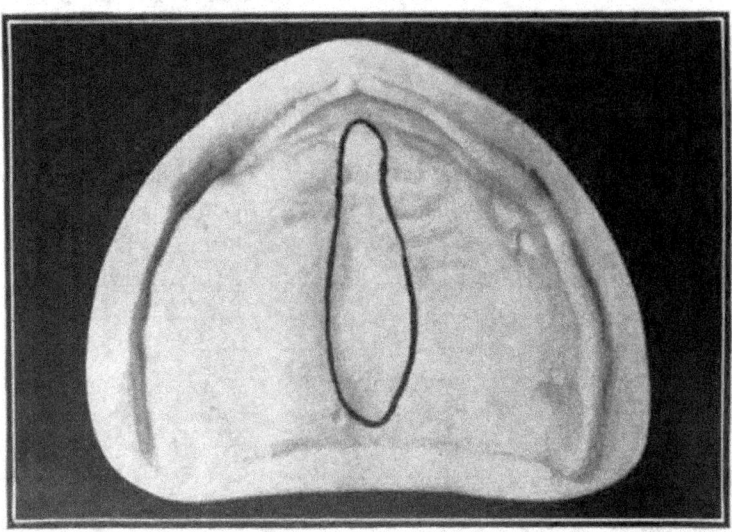

FIGURE 8.—Area to be relieved on upper model.

　b. The dental technician may prepare the areas indicated by the dental officer to be relieved by burnishing on the cast one or more layers of Nos. 40, 50, or 60 tinfoil which has been cut to fit the area for that particular case. As there can be no standard size and shape, the tinfoil must be cut for each case. The hardest areas are covered most thickly, but the thickness of the relief area should never be carried to the extent of creating a suction chamber, as in time this space would fill with hypertrophied tissue, thus defeating the purpose for which it was made. If tinfoil is unavailable, two or three layers of lead foil from X-ray films may be used in the same manner (fig. 8).

　28. Trial denture base.—Since a denture must fit the mouth accurately, it is first made on a trial base, such as wax, or other material which can be easily molded. This material should be of sufficient strength to hold its shape while the denture is tried in the mouth. Baseplate is preferable to wax as a trial denture base, however, because it holds its shape better and is not easily distorted by the temperature of the mouth. Procedure of adapting baseplate to cast is as follows:

　a. Pass the baseplate through the flame several times until it shows signs of wilting. Do not heat it too much as this will melt or burn the material (fig. 9).

b. Place the softened baseplate over the upper cast and adapt the palatal portion closely to the cast by pressing lightly with the fingers. Reheat the baseplate when necessary and continue adapting it over the alveolar border and over the buccal and labial surfaces (fig. 10).

c. Avoid buckling or creasing of the baseplate.

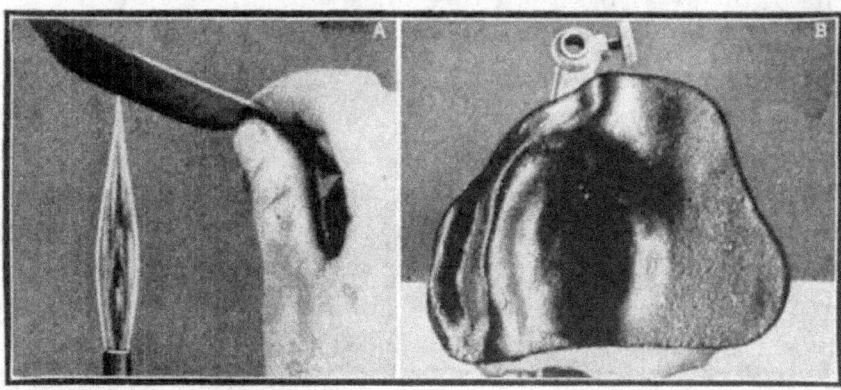

FIGURE 9. FIGURE 10.

d. Heat the partially adapted baseplate, and using plate shears trim away the surplus extending beyond the outer edges of the extension on the cast made by the carding wax rim in the boxing process. This is illustrated by *C* in figure 11.

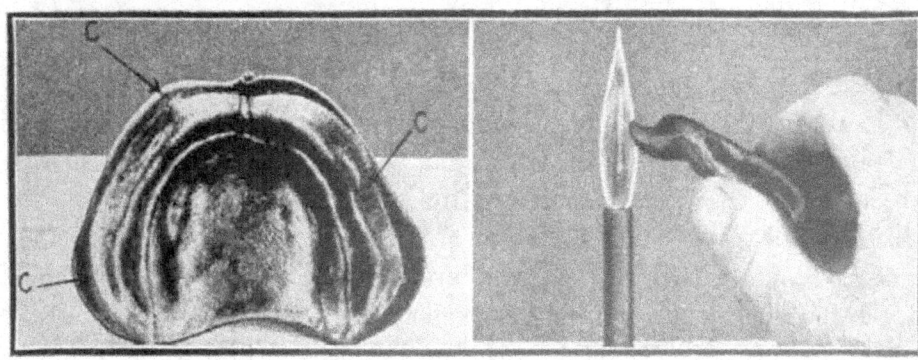

FIGURE 11. FIGURE 12.

e. Heat the baseplate which rests on the extension of the cast material by passing it once through the flame and folding the heated portion upon the buccal and labial surfaces by pressure, as shown in figure 13, and continue to the finished form, shown on the right side in figure 14. The folded portion is not heated enough to fuse with the baseplate against which it is folded. Fold the extension across the heel in the same manner. The margins thus shaped must conform to the muscle trim margins of the impression and constitute a valuable reenforcement of the baseplate.

f. Chill the baseplate with cold water and then carefully remove from the cast.

g. In lower casts adapt the trial baseplate material over the highest part of the alveolar ridge in the anterior region of the cast and work backward toward the heels. Treat the lingual, buccal, and labial margins of the lower baseplate the same as the upper.

h. If the trial baseplate should be broken, it may be repaired by placing the broken pieces on the cast with the edges together and fusing with a hot wax spatula. Melt some of the baseplate material in a flame and drop it over the break. Smooth the surface.

i. In partial cases, after adapting the baseplate to the palate and alveolar ridges, heat the material in the region of the plaster teeth and remove with a hot spatula or shears. This material should be removed to within $\frac{1}{32}$ inch from the gum margins of the plaster teeth, and the edges of the baseplate smoothed with a file.

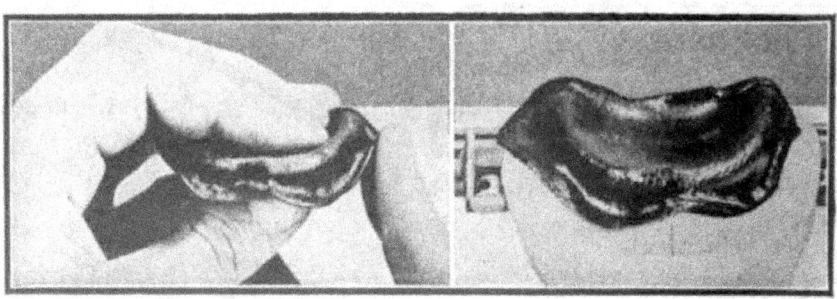

FIGURE 13.   FIGURE 14.

j. In partial lowers, it is necessary to reenforce the baseplate extending about the teeth by imbedding a hot wire or paper clip in the baseplate and smoothing the surface with a hot spatula.

29. Biteplates.—The mandible or lower jaw is movable, and is attached to the skull by two movable joints, giving it a hingelike motion. However, this is not a fixed motion as the jaw may also be moved in other directions within limits. In a mouth with natural teeth in place, the occlusal surfaces of these teeth act as guides which permit the jaws to come together in a rest or centric position. When the teeth are gone this relationship is missing. Therefore it is necessary to construct biteplates which will help the dental officer in reestablishing this relationship. Since the dental technician does not see the patient, he can only approximate the required size and shape of the biteplates.

a. Mark on the cast in a place where it can be seen, with the trial denture base in place, a line designating the crest of the alveolar ridge. This is for future reference in setting up the artificial teeth.

b. Soften a sheet of basewax by passing it over a flame several times, and fold it along its lesser length into a tight roll.

c. Bend the wax roll to the approximate shape of the alveolar ridge of the cast.

d. Replace the trial baseplate on the cast and attach the roll of wax, sealing it with a hot spatula.

e. Using a template or any flat surface, press the wax to the desired height. This is usually about 10 to 13 millimeters in height from the anterior portion of the alveolar ridge, and less in the molar region.

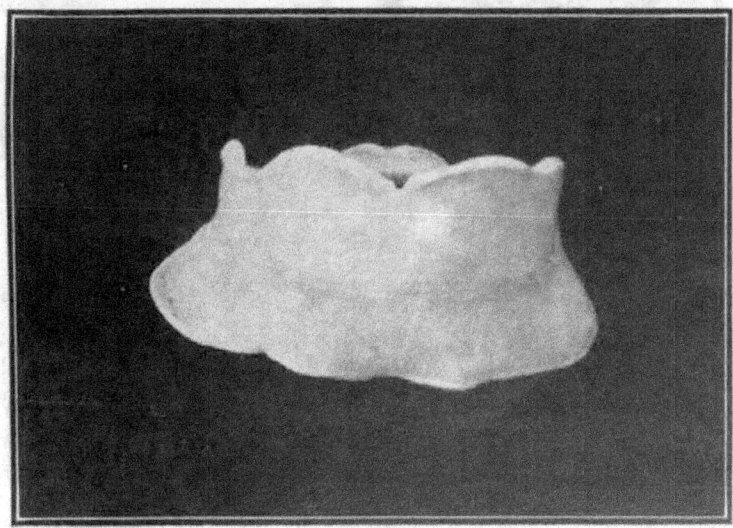

FIGURE 15.

f. With a knife and a hot spatula, trim the sides of the baseplate to a width of not more than 8 millimeters.

g. Add melted wax where necessary to fill in spaces between the wax roll and the baseplate on the buccal, labial, and lingual surfaces.

h. In partial cases be sure that the biteplate does not interfere with the teeth on the cast and cut the wax roll to fit the alveolar ridge where the teeth are missing, extending the wax about $1/16$ inch above the teeth of the cast but not covering the teeth.

i. Square up the sides and angles of the biteplate, making certain that it conforms to the cast and that it is directly over the crest of the alveolar ridge.

j. Polish the biteplate with wet cotton (fig. 15).

30. Mounting casts on articulator.—The cast or casts, with the biteplates constructed, are returned to the dental officer, who records the relationship of the patient's lower jaw to the upper jaw. This is known as "taking the bite." This established, the casts and biteplates come back to the dental technician ready to be placed on the arti ulator. The articulator used in the Army dental service is known as the Gysi simplex articulator, which simulates the movements of the jaw and has the plane of the condyle paths set at 30°. The procedure in mounting casts is as follows:

  a. Attach the biteplates to the casts with wax at several points.

  b. Place the casts in water until all bubbling has ceased.

  c. Place the incisor guide pin in the sleeve of the upper extension arm, keeping the top of the pin level with the top of the sleeve.

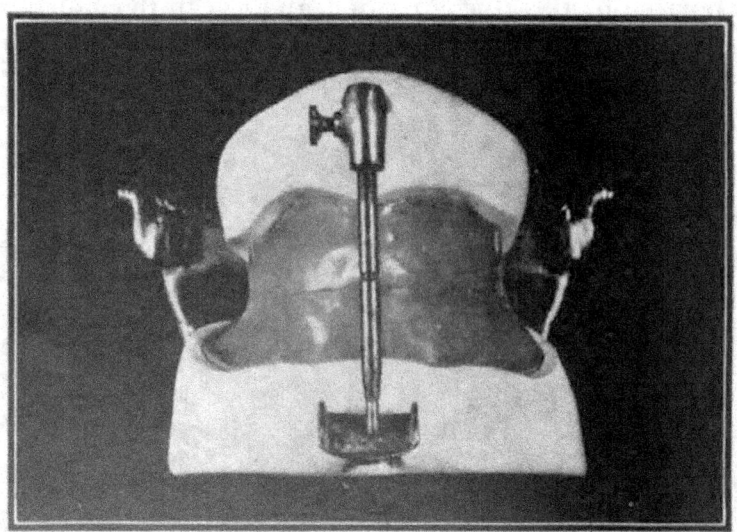

FIGURE 16.

  d. Place the incisal guide on the pin, with the setscrew in the depression of the pin and the point directed backward to the median line.

  e. Extend the median line mark on the front of the upper cast or bite rim vertically upward to the top of the cast. Make a similar vertical mark on the rear of the cast, starting from the median line of the palate. Draw a straight line across the cast connecting these two lines.

  f. Place an elastic band about the setscrew on the incisor guide point and in the notches on the outer sides of the vertical part of the frame. This line, as given by the elastic band, will establish the approximate occlusal plane.

  g. Place three small pieces of wax or moldine in a tripod arrangement on the lower extension arm, and force the lower cast down over these pieces until the occlusal plane of the biteplate is level with the elastic band, and the median line of the biteplate touches the tip of the incisor guide. Adjust the casts so that the median line of the upper cast is directly below the median line of the upper extension arm.

h. Attach the upper cast to the upper extension arm with plaster and allow to set. Then invert the articulator and attach the lower cast to the lower extension arm in the same manner.

i. Allow plaster to set and trim off all excess plaster (fig. 16).

j. Carefully separate the biteplates and remove the biteplates from the casts.

31. Selecting artificial teeth.—Before taking up the technique of setting the teeth, to which stage the case has been brought, consideration will be given to the question of selecting artificial teeth, of vital importance to both the efficiency and appearance of artificial dentures. In selecting artificial teeth, the two principal requirements to be considered are appearance, which includes form, proportion, and shade, and mechanics such as the length of bite and ridgelap necessary to the proper adaptation of the teeth to the ridges. These two factors are so often dependent upon each other that any apparent antagonism between them calls for judgment in making the necessary compromise. It may be stated as a safe rule to follow, that whenever the mechanical requirements interfere with the final appearance, the mechanics should be sacrificed as much as possible. While this may be questioned by some authorities, experience proves that appearance is the most important factor with the patient and many dentures which are mechanically perfect are unsatisfactory because they do not "look right."

32. Requirements of tooth forms.—Briefly, all teeth must correspond or harmonize in form and contour with the form and contour of the face which "frames" them in order to blend into the individuality of the person wearing them and insure the most pleasing effect. There are three typal forms of faces: square, tapering, and ovoid. These forms are further modified by an admixture of the elements of two or more of these typal forms. There are likewise the same typal forms of teeth. Whenever the face forms and tooth forms correspond and harmonize, the effect is good. To the extent that the teeth differ in form with faces, there is a disharmony which is displeasing in degree. For instance, when square teeth are framed in an ovoid face, the effect is unpleasant and the teeth are conspicuous, whereas when ovoid teeth are framed with an ovoid face the effect is pleasing in that the teeth do not seem to obtrude; they "belong" with the face. Tooth shade, form, and approximate size are always selected by the dental officer to conform with the requirement of the individual case, and such instructions should be followed as closely as mechanically possible. In the selection of teeth for partial cases the teeth should be of such size that after they have been contoured to the adjoining clasps or teeth they will completely fill the edentulous area.

TM 8-225
33   MEDICAL DEPARTMENT

33. **Arranging upper anteriors.**—*a.* Remove the upper bow from the articulator. Procure an occlusal plane or a flat piece of wood or aluminum 2½ inches square, and use it as shown in the illustration to take the place of the occlusal surface of the lower bite rim (**fig. 17**)

b. Before waxing the upper central in place, try for mechanical suit

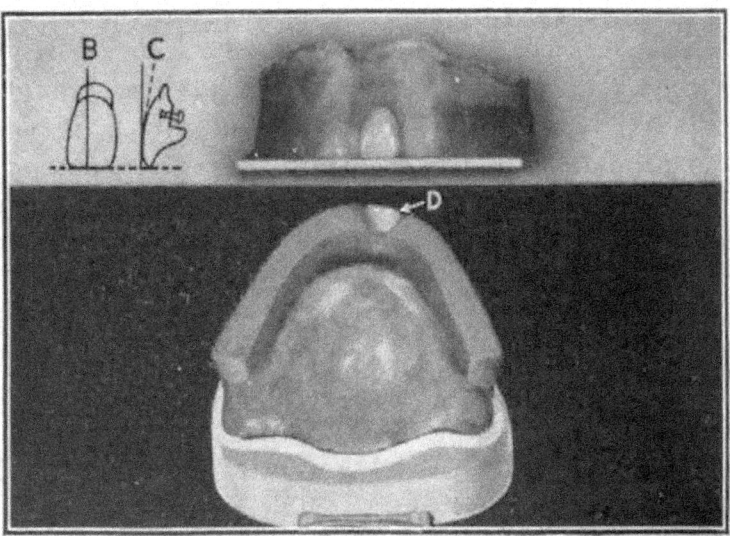

FIGURE 17.

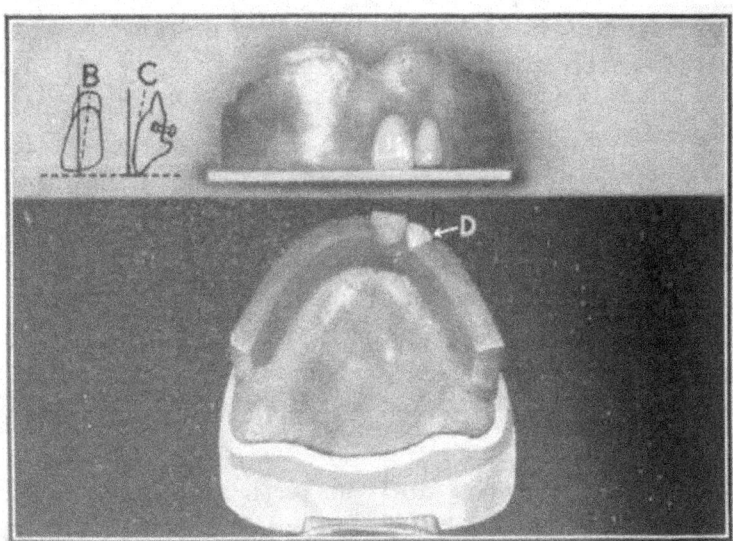

FIGURE 18.

ability. If necessary carve away the baseplate under the tooth or grind the ridgelap, or both, so that the tooth will not rest directly against the cast. The long axis of the upper central should be vertical when seen from the front and inclined downward and forward when seen from the side, as in *B* and *C*, figure 17. The incisal edge is in

36

contact with the occlusal plane. The upper centrals are not set at right angles to the median line, but the distal angles are inclined slightly backward and begin the curvature of the tooth row to follow the contour of the bite rim.

c. Cut a space through the upper bite rim for the upper lateral and try it in place as the central was tried. Set it so that the incisal edge is about 3/4 millimeter above the level of the occlusal plane and so that the long axis is inclined as in *B* and *C*, figure 18. This downward and forward inclination of the vertical axis of the upper laterals results in making the neck of this tooth less prominent than that of the upper central. This depression will be found very valuable when giving expression to the teeth. The incisal edges of the laterals are set to maintain the curvature established by the incisal edge of the upper bite rim, as shown at *D*.

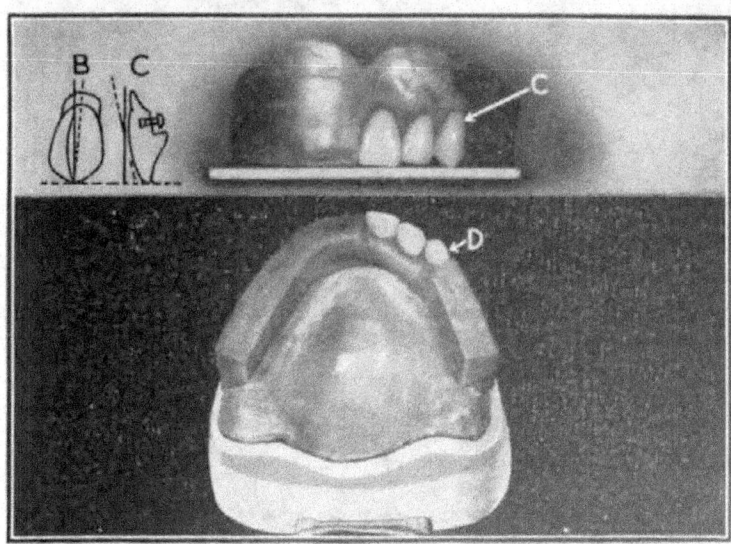

FIGURE 19.

d. Cut a space clear through the upper bite rim to receive the upper cuspid. Try the tooth for length as the central and lateral were tried. Set the tooth so that its tip just touches the occlusal plane and its long axis is inclined as shown in *B* and *C* and at the edge of the tooth continue the curve of the bite rim as shown at *D*, figure 19. The labial ridge of the cuspid is properly the dividing line between the labial and buccal sections of the ridge. The labial surface mesial to the ridge faces the lip and maintains the general curvature established by the central and lateral. The surface distal to this ridge faces the cheek and begins the curvature characteristic of the bicuspids and molars. The effect of setting the cuspids in this position is to carry the distal angles farther inward toward the median line. When the cuspids are set in this way, only the mesial aspect can be seen from the front. This permits the use of teeth large enough for the mouth, without their appearing too large. The esthetic effect of this arrangement is greatly enhanced by the natural shading of the teeth in the set and gives prominence to the neck or cervical third of both cuspids.

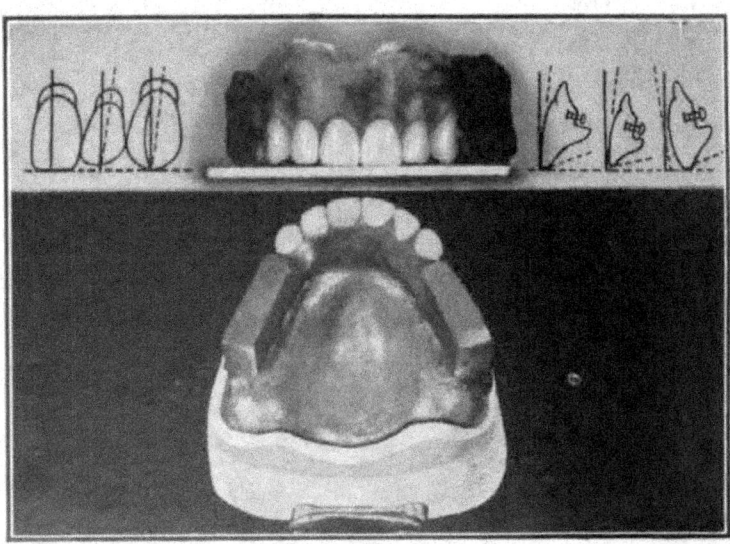

Figure 20.

e. When the central, lateral, and cuspid of one side have been set, set the central, lateral, and cuspid on the other side in the same manner (fig. 20).

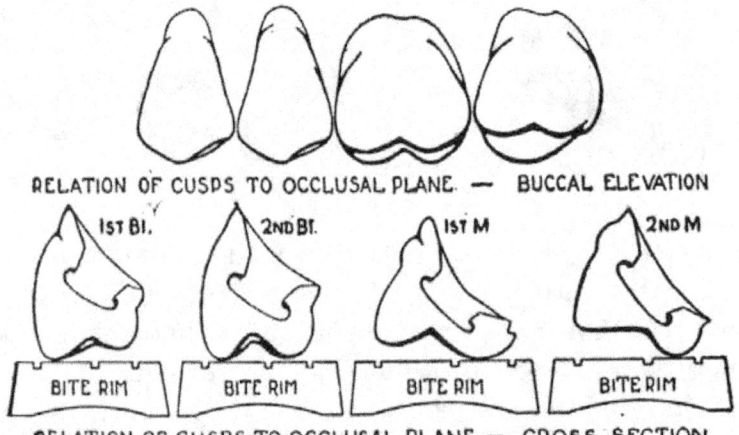

Figure 21.

34. **Arranging upper posteriors.**—a. Having determined the type of arch, the upper bicuspids and molars are set with their vertical axes in the lines shown in figure 21.

b. The buccal cusp of the upper first bicuspid touches the occlusal surface of the lower trial plate, but the lingual cusp does not quite touch. Both cusps of the upper second bicuspids touch the wax (fig. 22). The buccal cusps of the upper first molar are elevated about a millimeter above the wax to begin the compensating curve formed by the buccal cusp of both upper molars. The lingual cusps of the second molars are in contact with the opposing trial plate, but the buccal cusps are elevated about 2 millimeters above the wax. They continue the compensating curve which the buccal cusps of the first molars began.

c. It is necessary, while establishing these relations, to secure such positions of the teeth over the ridge as to give the dentures maximum

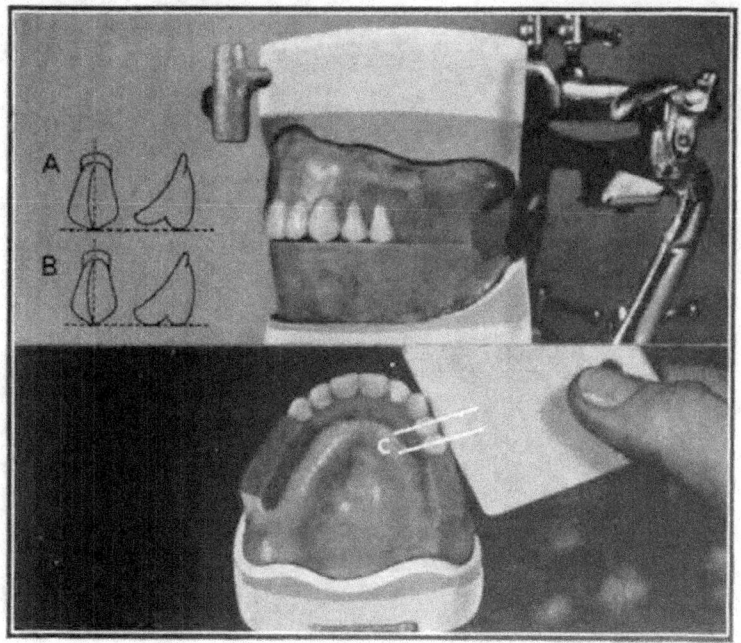

Figure 22.

stability and efficiency. Fit each posterior tooth to its position before waxing it in place, as the anteriors were fitted. Make sure that each tooth is short enough so that there is a free space of at least a millimeter between it and the baseplate. Cut a strip ½ inch wide along the side of a sheet of baseplate wax and soften one end of it in the flame. Detach a small portion and form it into a cone. Soften the end of the cone in the flame and force it about the pins or into the recess in the diatoric tooth. Using the tooth as a handle, soften the other end of the cone and press it upon the ridge with the tooth in approximately the correct position. Close the articular so that the incisor guide pin comes into contact with the incisor guide incline. Adjust the teeth so that the center of the longitudinal groove is over the **front-to-back** line on the occlusal surface of the lower bite rim.

The buccal cusp of the upper first bicuspid should touch the occlusal surface of the lower bite; the lingual cusp should be raised about ½ millimeter above that rim. When the tooth is first placed, the long axis of the tooth, as seen from the buccal, should be vertical, as shown at A in figure 22. This may be slightly modified in establishing articulation. The second bicuspid should be set like the first except that both cusps touch the opposing bite rim, as shown at B in figure 22. Rotate both bicuspids upon their long axis so that the occlusal surfaces are inclined as shown by the lines in C, figure 22. With the straightedge of the occlusal plane, test the position of the buccal

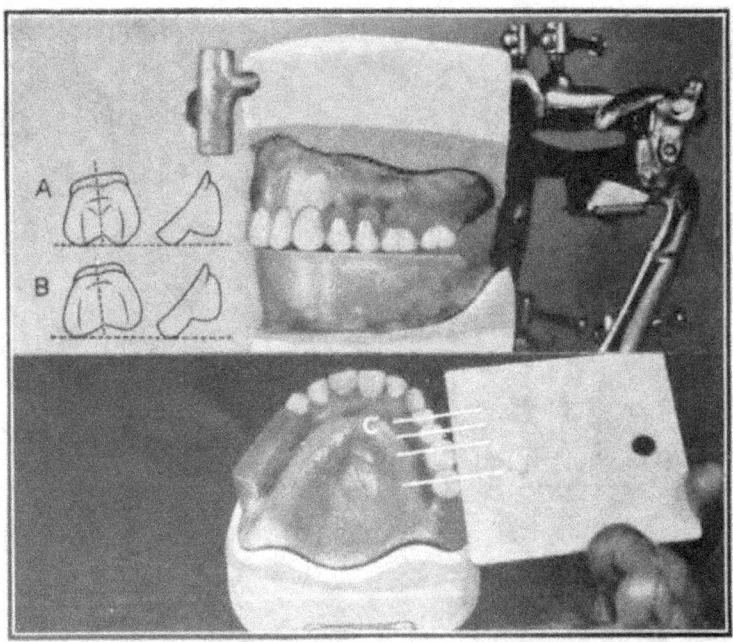

FIGURE 23.

surface of the bicuspid in relation to the cuspids. When these teeth are in proper relation for the average case, the straightedge should touch the buccal surfaces of all three teeth.

d. Attach the upper first molar to the ridge as the bicuspids were attached. The long axis of this tooth, when seen from the buccal, is inclined downward and backward as shown at A, figure 23. Only the mesio-lingual cusp of this tooth should touch the occlusal surface of the opposing bite, the disto-lingual cusp being slightly raised and the buccal cusp being raised about ¾ millimeter out of contact, as shown in A, figure 23. This arrangement produces the average compensating curve. When a greater curvature is required, the distal cusps should be elevated more. The tooth should be rotated upon its long axis as shown at C in figure 23.

e. The upper second molar is now placed in position, with its lingual cusps lightly touching the occlusal plane and the buccal cusp raised about 1½ millimeters out of contact as shown in *B*, figure 23. If a greater curvature is desired, the lingual cusp should be elevated out of contact and the buccal cusps elevated in a corresponding degree. The long axis, seen from the buccal, is inclined downward and backward more than was the first molar.

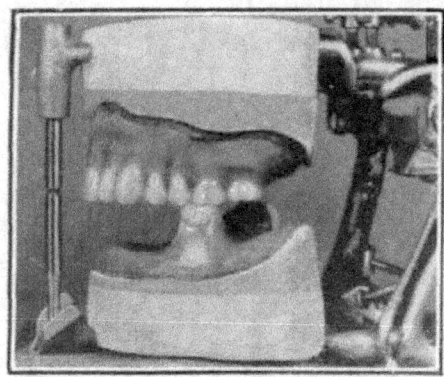

Figure 24.

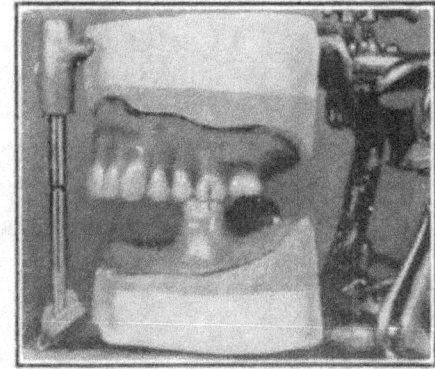

Figure 25.

35. Arranging lower first molar.—Apply a cone of wax to a lower first molar. Open the articulator and attach the molar to the ridge in approximately the correct position, but too high. Close the

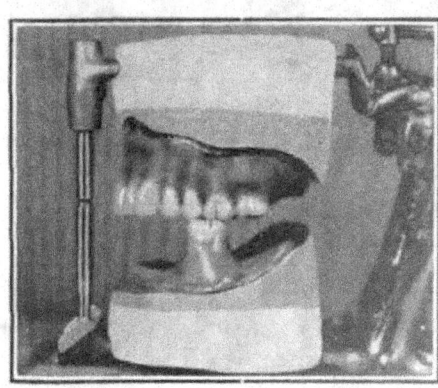

Figure 26.

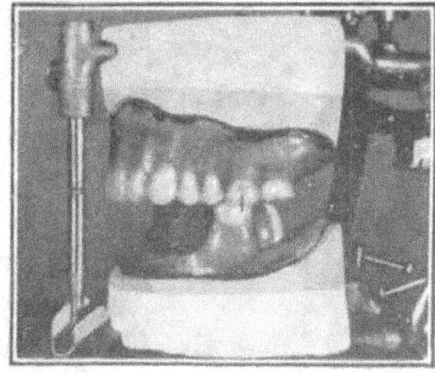

Figure 27.

articulator, forcing the molar toward the ridge. Guide it to correct occlusal relations with the uppers as in figure 24. Wax the molar firmly in position. Move the articulator so as to throw this molar into working bite with the uppers, as in figure 25. A black line has been drawn along the buccal ridge of the middle cusp of the lower molar. It should be continuous with the black line in the buccal groove of the upper molar. The break in the line in figure 26 shows that the lower molar is too far forward for articulation. Figures 24 and 26 show that teeth may be in good position for occlusion without being in position to articulate. In figure 25 the lower molar has been moved backward so that the black line is continuous with the line on the upper, in working bite, but the buccal cusps do not interdigitate with the upper cusps. Errors of this kind can usually be corrected by depressing the buccal cusps of the upper molar, but in this case the steep descending inclination of the condyle path, with the slight lateral inclination, necessitated grinding the teeth to a deeper bite. With a fine-grit, inverted cone stone the mesial marginal ridge of the upper molar and the distal marginal ridge of the lower molar were ground until they could be properly interdigitated. In figure 27 the molars are shown in working bite after deepening the sulci by grinding has been completed and the lower molar reset to proper contact with the upper. The space between the upper

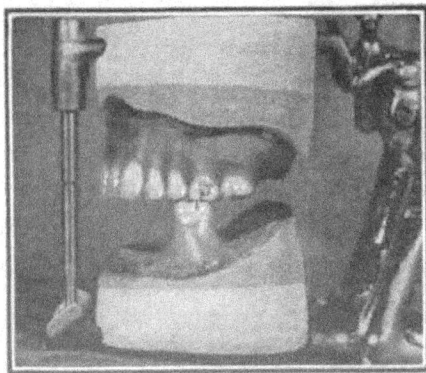 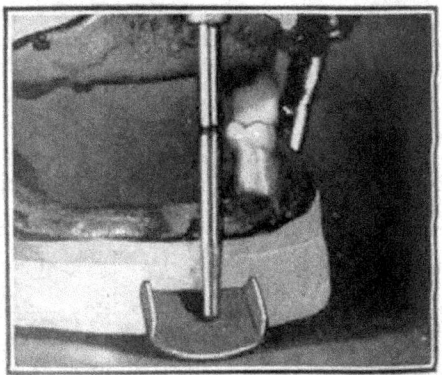

FIGURE 28.   FIGURE 29.

second bicuspid and the lower molar in figure 25 has been decreased by deepening the bite of the molars and raising the lower molar. The lower first molar in figure 28 is in the same position on the ridge that it occupied in figure 27, but the articulator has been moved so as to throw this side into balancing relation. The triangular ridge of the mesio-lingual cusp of the upper molar should slide in the disto-buccal groove of the lower molar, but cusp and groove are separated by a slight space. A defect of this kind can usually be corrected by depressing the lingual cusp of the upper molar until contact is established and waxing the upper firmly in that position. It may be necessary to rotate either the upper or the lower on its vertical axis until the cusp works smoothly in the groove. Examine the working bite articulation from the lingual, as shown in figure 30. The slight prominence of the mesio-lingual cusp of the lower molar, indicated by the arrow, prevents correct relations in the working bite. Grind this away with the inverted cone stone, being careful to maintain the original inclination of the cusp planes. Do not grind a flat surface on the tip of the cusp. The upper and lower molars, in occlusion,

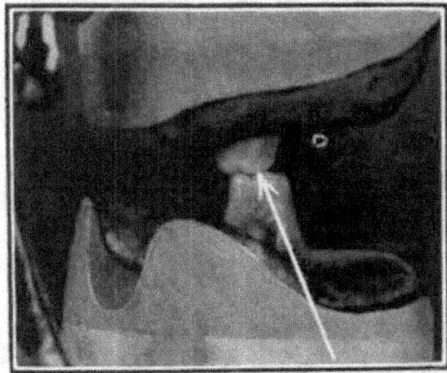
FIGURE 30.

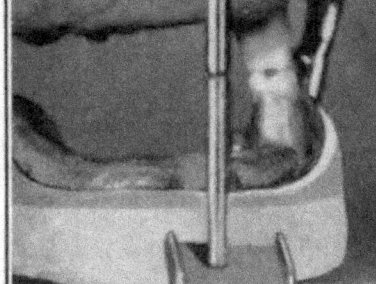
FIGURE 31.

should mesh as in figure 29. The buccal cusp of the lower should fill the V-shaped longitudinal groove between the lingual and buccal

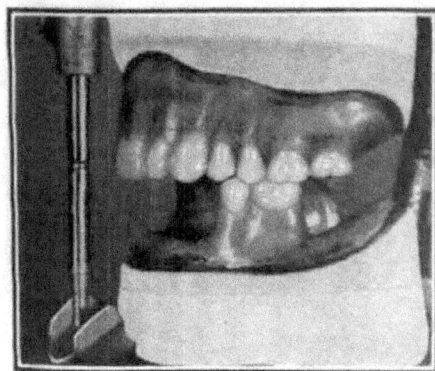
FIGURE 32.

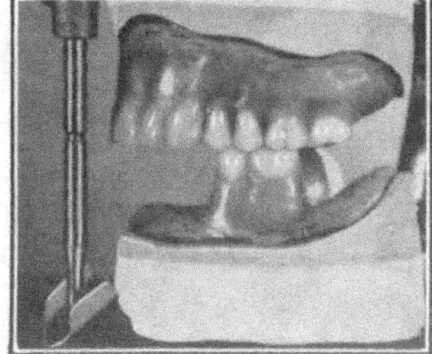
FIGURE 33.

cusps of the upper. The lingually inclined plane of the lower buccal cusp should be in contact with the buccally inclined plane of the lingual cusp. Figure 31 shows the relation of the upper and lower molars in working bite.

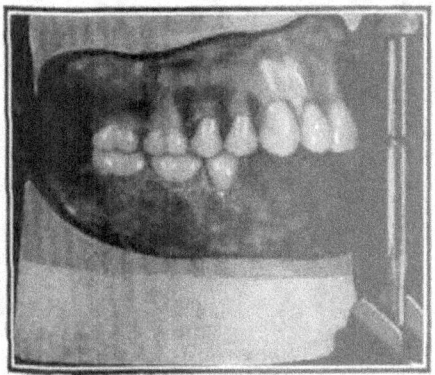
FIGURE 34.

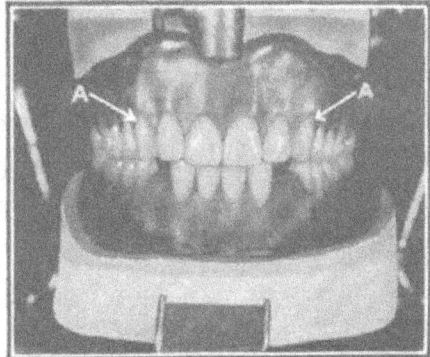
FIGURE 35.

36

36. Arranging lower second bicuspid.—*a.* After completing the articulation of the upper and lower molars for the case here illustrated, the distal marginal ridge of the upper second bicuspid was ground in the manner described for the first molars until the buccal cusp of the bicuspid could be brought down in contact with the buccal cusp of the lower molar when in working-bite relation.

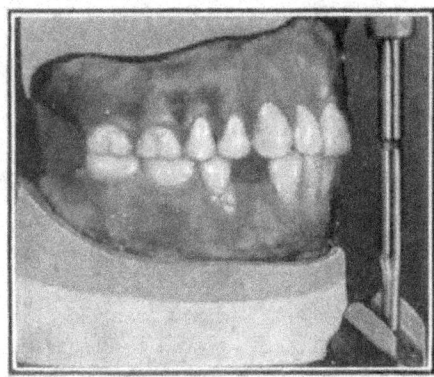

FIGURE 36.

The tooth was then examined from the lingual and adjusted to mesh properly with the lower molar in working bite. Attach a cone of wax to the neck of the lower second bicuspid and place it on the ridge in the manner described for the molar and with a spatula press it into approximate occlusion with the upper second bicuspid. Move the articulator so as to test the articulation in working bite, which is shown in figure 33.

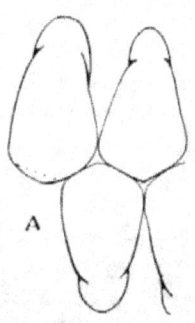 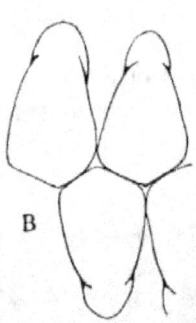 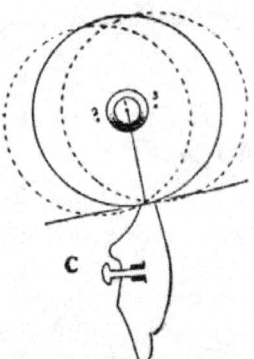

A. Before grinding in correct relation to working bite.

B. After grinding.

C. Relation of center of stone to the long axis of cuspid for grinding bucco-lingual pitch on the facet. Solid circle, center 1, shows correct position; dotted circles, centers 2 and 3, show incorrect positions.

FIGURE 37.—Mesial facet of upper cuspids.

b. The space between the lower second bicuspid and the molar in figure 33 will exist whenever the conditions of the case necessitate a compensating curve of more than average steepness. The existence of such spaces compensates in part for the shrinkage of rubber in vulcanizing and reduces the liability of error from the teeth being forced into improper contact through that shrinkage. Occlude and articulate the lower second molar as shown in figure 34. Set the lower second bicuspid for occlusion and then for articulation by the methods described. Arrange the lower molars and the second bicuspid of the opposite side, using the same technique. Set the lower anteriors to approximate positions to determine whether they meet the requirements of the case as to width and length. If insufficient space exists between the lower bicuspid to permit setting the lower anteriors because of irregularities in the alinement of the upper anteriors, additional space may be made by grinding the distal side of the lower cuspids or the mesial side of the lower first molar.

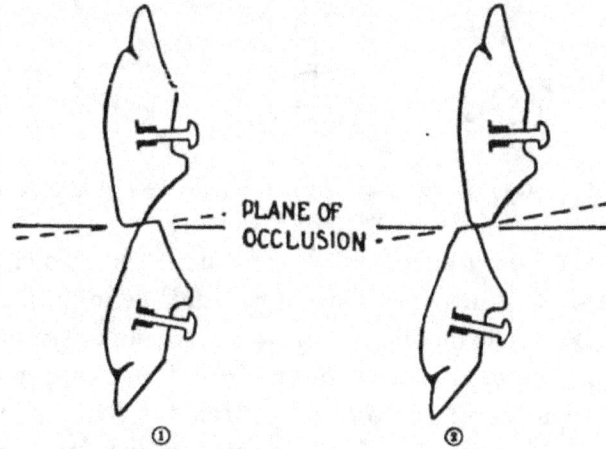

FIGURE 38.—Cuspids in rest and beginning of working-bite relation, dotted line indicating proper bucco-lingual inclination for these cusp facets.

c. If sufficient space cannot be provided by such grinding, select lower anteriors of the next smaller size in the same form.

37. Arranging lower anteriors.—The roots of the lower centrals and laterals are parallel, but those of the lower cuspids diverge strongly as will be pointed out later when the lower cuspid is articulated. The lower centrals slope strongly outward from the neck to the incisal edge. This prevents the overfullness of the gums so common to lower dentures. The lower laterals slope outward considerably less than do the centrals. This is shown in figure 39.

38. Arranging cuspids.—*a.* The upper lateral adjoining the cuspid should be removed from its place without heating the wax, so that it can be easily replaced. This will facilitate articulating the lower cuspid.

   b. Set the lower cuspid in position and grind the mesio-distal inclination of the distal half of the cutting edge to be parallel to the inclination of the cutting edge of the mesial half of the upper cuspid as in figure 36. The facet on the mesial slope on the upper cuspid is to be ground to the lingual inclination shown by the outline in figure 37, so that a straightedge placed in contact with the facet will touch the wax at the mesio-lingual cusp of the first molar. Grind the facet on the distal slope of the cutting edge of the lower cuspid to a labial inclination which is the complement of the lingual slope of the upper cuspid with which it occludes as shown in figure 38. The

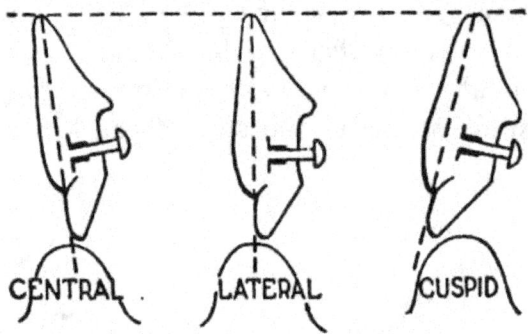

FIGURE 39.—Relation of lower cuspids and incisors to ridge, and average inclination for long axes.

inclination of the long axis of the lower cuspid is also shown in figure 38. In figure 38① the complementary inclination of the facets on the cutting edges of the cuspids is shown with the cuspids in occlusion. In figure 38②, the cuspids are shown in articulation with the lower about to begin the return from an extreme lateral excursion. The complementary inclinations of the facets make it possible for the cuspids to remain in contact throughout these movements. This form of articulation by the cuspids is very important in maintaining the stability of the dentures and in protecting the upper laterals from breakage. If the lower cuspids are set to too deep an under bite, the dentures are almost sure to be tipped out of position by improper cuspid contacts; the force of the closure will be brought upon the thin-edged laterals which are not fitted to stand it, and they will be broken from the plate. This form of improper contact is very apt to occur in finished dentures unless guarded against and is disastrous.

   c. Replace the upper lateral but do not attach it. Move the articulator to produce the working and balancing relations and grind the mesial edge of the lower cuspid so that it clears the slope on the distal angle of the upper lateral. The upper laterals and the lower cuspids should not come into contact in any movement of the jaw. The facet on the cutting edge of the upper lateral should incline upward and backward more than that on the edge of the cuspid. When this facet has been ground, articulate the lower lateral with it. Do not grind facets on the cutting edges of the lower incisors. Grind facets on the edges of the upper centrals and articulate the lower centrals with them. The lower incisors should be set with the necks directly over the ridge and the long axis of the teeth should be inclined as is shown in figure 39.

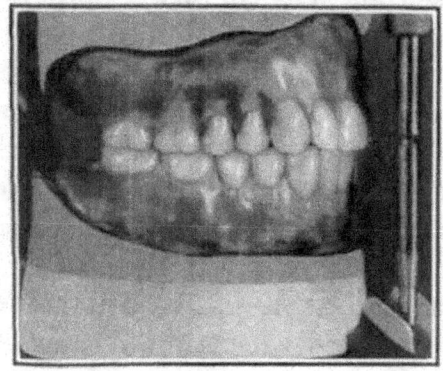

FIGURE 40.

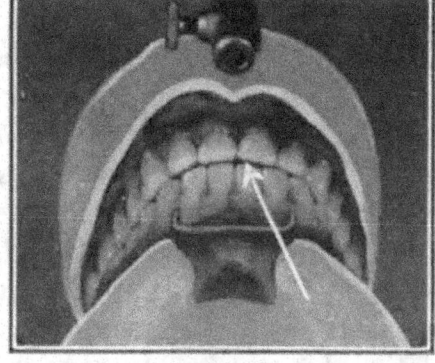

FIGURE 41.

39. Arranging lower first bicuspid.—The lower first bicuspid is the last tooth to be placed. It is articulated in the same manner as the second bicuspid. If the indicated space is not adequate to accommodate the lower first bicuspid, the mesio-distal width of the tooth is reduced by grinding. Never crowd the lower anterior teeth out of position and off the ridge in order to place this tooth. Figure 40 shows the tooth in position.

40. Incising bite.—*a.* Before the teeth are tried in the mouth, hold the articulator in the incising position and slightly alter the arrangement of the incisors and cuspids if necessary so that they will come into proper contact. The upper centrals should touch the lower centrals. The upper laterals may, in certain arrangements, touch the lower laterals, but they should not touch the lower cuspids. Most instances of broken laterals not due to careless handling have been found to be due to a cuspid striking the lateral in the incising or the working bite. The lower cuspids should touch the upper cuspids but not the upper laterals in masticating movements. Figure 41 shows the average overjet of the upper anteriors over the lower teeth.

b. When the lower is in central occlusion the lower incisors and possibly the lower cuspids should not be in contact. The lower incisors should not be allowed to support the dentures in lateral protrusive movements but should share this strain with the bicuspids and the cuspids. The pressure on the cuspids should be heavier than on the upper laterals or the lower incisors. The danger of breaking the incisors during mastication will be eliminated if the foregoing instructions are observed and the errors seen in the finished denture are corrected by grinding with a stone while the dentures are examined for these contacts in the mouth. The lower first bicuspid should be in contact with the upper cuspid which acts as a protector for the upper lateral and prevents the incisors from receiving any excessive strain. The tip of the cusp of the lower second bicuspid may touch the tip of the upper first bicuspid cusp but this is not essential. The tip of the upper second bicuspid should come into contact with the mesio-buccal cusp of the lower first molar. The lingual cusps of the bicuspids and molars also come into contact in the incising-bite relation. Occasionally the lingual cusps will touch so heavily that the buccal cusps cannot come into contact. If any cusp rides so heavily on an opposing cusp as to prevent the teeth from coming into the proper relation with their antagonists, a little careful grinding will correct the trouble.

41. **Balancing bite.**—The depth of this bite is the distance the lower teeth on the balancing side move vertically to maintain balancing relations between the dentures during articulation. It is much greater than the depth of the working bite, because the steep lingual inclines of the lower buccal cusps articulate with the steep inclines of the lingual cusps of the upper teeth, and because the lower cusps often travel directly across the steepest parts of the upper cusps instead of following the sulci.

42. **Central dental laboratory assortment of new Trubyte teeth.**—The following charts give the assortment of teeth chosen for the central dental laboratories for shades and molds. The data given in *b* below assist in choosing teeth and matching the lower anteriors and posteriors with the upper anteriors. The shades of the New Hue and the new Trubyte teeth, as selected for Army use, are given below, with the corresponding shades for the old Trubyte teeth.

DENTAL TECHNICIANS

a. Shades.

New Hue	New Trubyte	Old Trubyte
63	40	5
66	41	6
67	43	7
77	46	9
81	49	14
69	52	15
79	55	16
83	57	20

b. Data.—(1) *Upper anteriors, 1×6.*—(a) *Square type.*

Mold No.	Width of central (mm)	Posteriors required	Lower anteriors required
115	8.5	34M—31L	25
117	9.5	34L—35L	27
123	7.5	30L—29L	33
124	8	32L—31L	34
126	9	34L—33L	36
133s	7.5	30M—29M	43s
134	8	32M—31M	44
135s	8.5	32L—31M	45s
136s	9	34M—33M	46s
155	8.5	32M—31M	34

TM 8-225
MEDICAL DEPARTMENT

(b) *Tapering type.*

Mold No.	Width of central (mm)	Posteriors required	Lower anteriors required
214	8	32L—31L	34
217	9.5	34L—35L	27
222	7	28S—29S	31
224	8	30L—31M	33
225s	8.5	32L—31L	45s
225	8.5	32L—31L	34
226s	9	34M—33L	46s
233	7.5	30M—29L	32
234	8	32L—31L	34
235	8.5	34M—31L	35
244	8	32L—31M	34
262	7	28L—29L	22
263	7.5	30L—29L	23
264	8	32L—31L	24
265	8.5	34L—31L	25
266	9	34L—33L	26
267	9.5	34L—35L	27
275	8.5	32L—31M	45

(c) *Ovoid type.*

Mold No.	Width of central (mm)	Posteriors required	Lower anteriors required
314	8	32L—31L	24
315	8.5	32L—31L	25
317	9.5	34L—35L	27
324	8	32L—31L	24
333	7.5	30L—29M	23
334	8	32L—31M	24
335	8.5	34M—31L	25
346	9	34L—33M	46

(2) *Lower anteriors, 1×6.*—Molds available: 22, 23, 24, 25, 26, 27, 31, 32, 33, 34, 35, 36, 43, 43s, 44, 45, 45s, 46, and 46s.

(3) *Upper and lower posteriors, 1×8.*—(*a*) *Regular.*—Molds available: 28S, 28M, 28L, 30S, 30M, 30L, 32S, 32M, 32L, 34S, 34M, 34L, and 32X.

(*b*) *Twenty degrees.*—Molds available: 29S, 29M, 29L, 31S, 31M, 31L, 33S, 33M, 33L, and 35L.

43. Debenture waxing.—After the teeth are arranged, the technician proceeds with the carving of the wax so that he has an exact duplicate of the finished denture. By this method the wax denture may be placed in the mouth and checked for appearance and mechanical efficiency by the dental officer, and if any changes are necessary, they can be made at this time. The procedure is as follows:

a. Add melted wax to the case in deficient areas, especially along the buccal and labial surfaces of the denture. This will later be

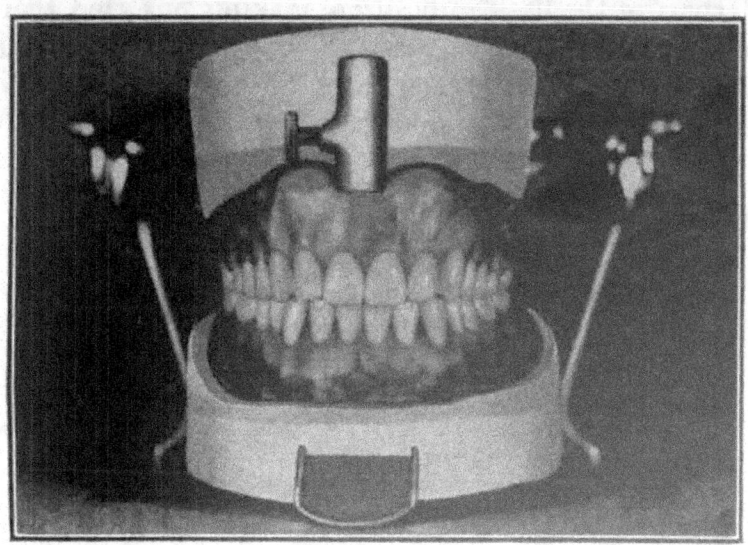

FIGURE 42.

carved so as to simulate the irregularities of the gum caused by the roots of the natural teeth.

b. With a knife or wax spatula, festoon all teeth at right angles to the long axis of the teeth. This should be carried to the necks of the teeth on the buccal, labial, and lingual surfaces. Do not festoon too deeply in the interproximal spaces between the teeth.

c. Smooth the entire surface of the wax by passing a flame quickly over the area. It may be further polished by rubbing with a piece of cotton while holding it under running cold water.

d. The waxed denture is now ready for try-in (fig. 42).

44. Denture flasking (full).—This is the process by which the wax or trial denture is started on a new series of procedures from which will emerge the finished denture. The denture base, after having been checked in the patient's mouth by the dental officer, is sealed to the cast and invested in a flask so as to retain the exact relationship of the teeth and preserve the space from which the wax will be eliminated so that it may be filled with dental rubber or some other material. The flasking process will maintain this space and relationship while the denture is being vulcanized or cured. The procedure is as follows:

a. Seal the waxed denture to the cast along its entire periphery and make sure that all the teeth are securely waxed in place.

b. Remove the models from the articulator.

c. Cut out the palate of the trial denture base and adapt one and one-half thicknesses of baseplate wax to the palate of the case.

d. Place the cast in the lower part of the flask. Then place the upper or counterpart of the flask in position, making sure that there is sufficient room in the flask for the case. Place the cover on the flask, making certain that the teeth do not touch the top of the flask. At least ¼ inch of space should be maintained.

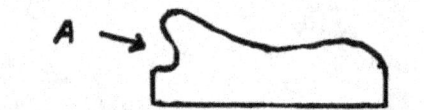

FIGURE 43.—Undercut (A) when cast is flasked level.

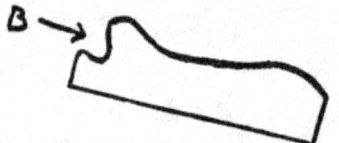

FIGURE 44.—Elimination of undercut (B) when cast is flasked at an angle.

e. Remove the cast from the flask and immerse in cold water for a few minutes until all bubbling ceases.

f. Make a plaster of paris mix of a heavy creamy consistency, and fill the lower portion of the flask to about two-thirds of its capacity. If the plaster is too thin it is difficult to control, and will extend upon the waxed surfaces.

g. If no undercuts are present on the cast, settle it in the plaster mix so that the occlusal plane of the teeth will be parallel with the bottom of the flask. If undercuts are present, as they sometimes are around the anterior region or the heels, it is necessary to place the cast in 3 plaster at such an angle so as to compensate for the undercut. For instance, if the anterior ridge is undercut, it is necessary to raise the anterior portion of the cast above the level of the heels (figs. 43 and 44).

h. Remove all excess plaster between the peripheral rim of the denture and the rim of the lower portion of the flask, smoothing the surface of the plaster.

i. Allow plaster to set until hard and then apply a little petrolatum or green soap to the surface of the plaster to act as a separating medium.

j. Set the upper portion of the flask in position.

k. Make a plaster mix and fill the upper portion of the flask, pouring the plaster carefully, and gently jarring the case so as to prevent inclusion of air bubbles.

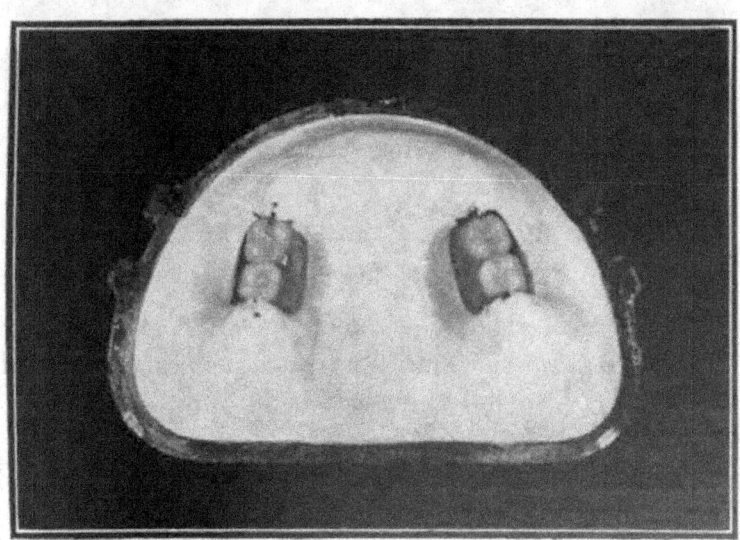

FIGURE 45.

l. Place the top of the flask in position and wipe off all excess plaster.

45. Denture flasking (partial).—*a.* (1) *Holding of clasps and framework to models upon separation.*—The first method to be described consists of flasking the denture similarly to that just described, but in addition, cutting off the remaining teeth from the cast to within 1/16 inch from the wax. This exposes all the clasps. When removing the plaster tooth from within a clasp, extreme caution should be exercised. It is often advisable to remove such teeth with a bur. After removal of the plaster tooth from the clasped area, any adjacent voids in the wax should be filled with wax. These clasps as well as any other metal parts such as lingual bars, etc., are then covered with plaster mix in the lower portion of the flask, leaving just the wax surfaces and artifical teeth exposed. From this point the flasking is carried out as given above (fig. 45).

(2) *Removal of clasp and framework from model upon separation.*—Another method of flasking partial dentures is frequently used,

especially in the acrylic resin cases that require tinfoiling. It consists of cutting off all the teeth from the model to within 1/16 inch from the wax. The exposed clasps, bars, etc., are then incorporated into the

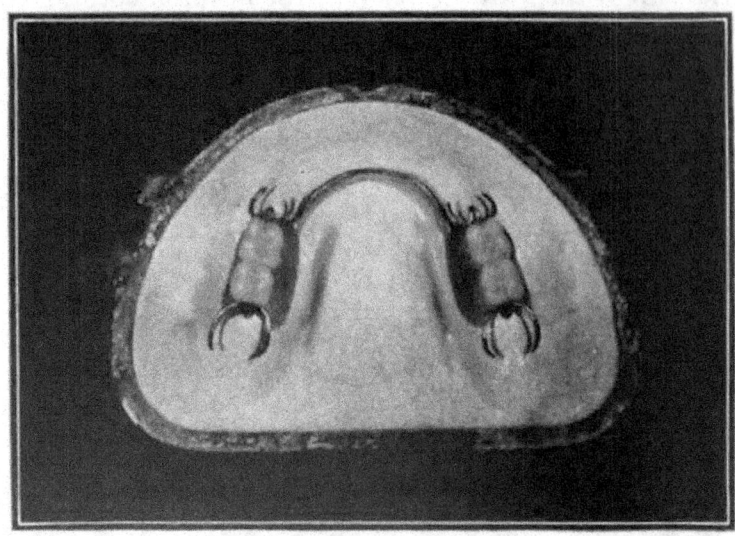

FIGURE 46.

upper portion of the flask instead of the lower. It is often advisable in the case of palatal and lingual bars to remove a portion of the cast from about the bar to insure their retention and more stable relationship when using this method. When the plaster in the upper half has set, the wax eliminated and the flask opened as described in the next step, the clasps, etc., will be pulled away from the model, but still will maintain their correct relationship (fig. 46).

  b. Either method of flasking may be used, depending upon the individual case under construction. In either method, prior to the pouring of the upper half of the flask, make doubly sure that all undercuts are eliminated in order to prevent fracture or irreparable damage to the models upon separation of the flask.

  46. **Packing the case.**—The case is now ready to be packed with any material that has been selected. Dental rubber or vulcanite and acrylic resin are the most satisfactory and the most commonly used. Therefore, only these materials will be discussed. All cases should be carefully packed with the right quantity of material. There is no reason for overpacking and thus inviting danger of breakage of the cast and the destruction of the occlusion of the teeth. The "dry" method of packing vulcanite cases is the most desirable.

  a. The pink gum rubber is cut into strips which are wide enough to cover the ridge lap of the teeth and extend to the border of the matrix. A narrow strip is then cut into small, triangular pieces which will fill the spaces between the teeth. The base rubber is cut into the desired size pieces for the lingual and hidden parts of the case. Pink rubber is used on the labial and buccal surfaces of the denture because it has a much more natural appearance. Base rubber is used on the palatal and hidden surfaces of the denture because it is much stronger and more durable than the pink rubber.

b. The lower part of the flask is placed in a heated oven and warmed throughout to a temperature of about 212°. It is then removed from the oven and placed on a towel which will serve as a heat retainer during the packing process.

c. Using suitable packing tools, carefully place the triangular pieces of rubber between the interproximal spaces of the teeth.

d. Fold a strip of dark rubber about ¼ inch wide along its greater length, and cut a piece long enough to fit from the first bicuspid region of one side to the first bicuspid region of the other. Insert this piece of rubber under the pins of the anterior teeth.

e. Pack the small square pieces of the dark rubber into each one of the diatoric openings of the posterior teeth (fig. 47).

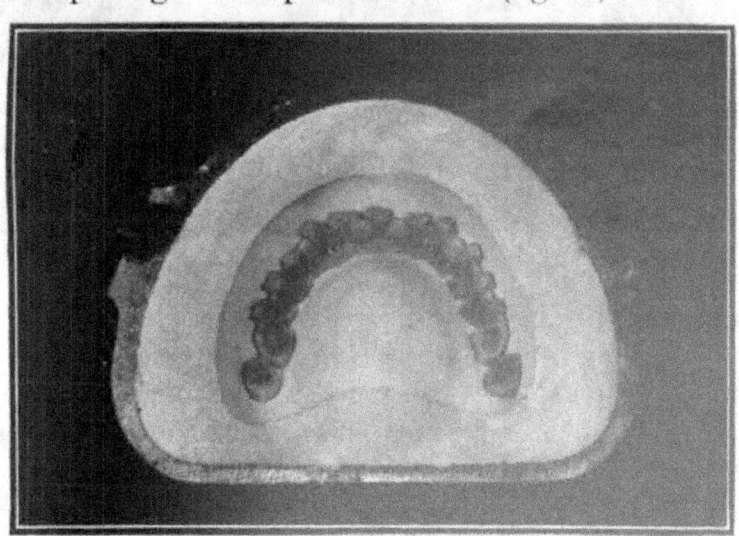

FIGURE 47.

f. Place two strips of the pink rubber, about ½ inch in width, one over the other, and lay them over the triangular pieces and the edge of the teeth along the buccal and labial surfaces from the median line to the region of the second molar. Place two more strips of the pink rubber in identical positions on the other side. These pink strips should extend from about 1 millimeter above the pins and diatoric openings to about 1 millimeter above the rim of the denture.

g. Place small strips of the dark rubber close against the pink rubber in the region of the buccal surface of the second molars.

h. Place additional strips of dark rubber against the bicuspids and molars on the palate.

i. Cover the remaining portion of the palate with the dark rubber, and add sufficient rubber over the entire surface to fill completely the space formerly occupied by the wax. It should be filled so that a little excess may be squeezed out around the edge of the denture when the flask is closed (fig. 48).

j. The lower denture is packed in a similar manner as the upper with the exception of having the tongue space instead of the palate. The lingual flanges of the lower denture are packed with the dark rub-

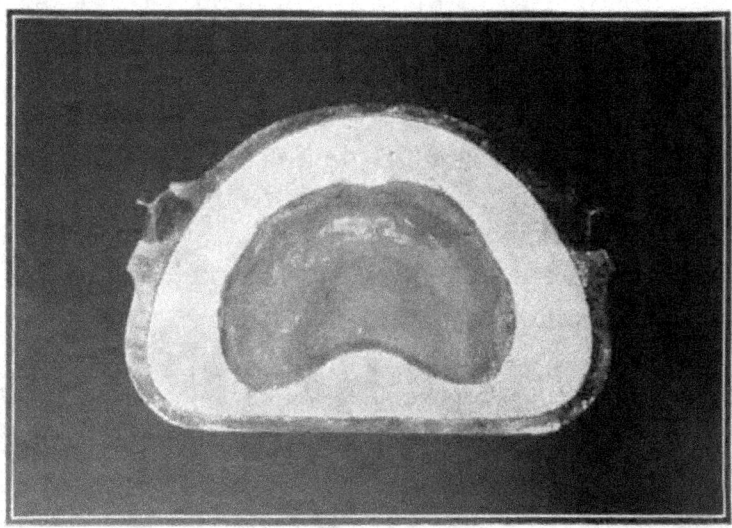

FIGURE 48.

ber, and are carried just 1 millimeter beyond the periphery of the denture. The tongue space is left free from rubber.

k. If much time has been consumed in packing the case and it has become cold before the packing operation is completed, it may be returned to the oven and reheated.

l. When the packing of the case has been completed, a piece of wet cellophane is laid over the entire lower half of the flask, and the two parts of the flask are then brought together.

m. Place the flask in a flask press and immerse both in a pan of boiling water for about 15 minutes. Remove from water and cautiously apply pressure with the screw. Too much pressure must not be applied in closing the flask.

n. The flask is removed from the press and opened. If too much rubber has been expressed, the excess is removed and the operation repeated.

o. If rubber is insufficient, add more and repeat the process (fig. 49).

p. Adapt a piece of wet cellophane to the cast before the final closing of the case. As the tissue surface of the completed denture is never polished, this step is necessary to insure a dense, smooth surface. Tinfoil may be adapted to the case in place of the cellophane, if desired.

47. Vulcanizing.—*a.* Fill the vulcanizer pot with warm water to a depth of 1 inch.

b. Place the flask clamp containing the flask in the vulcanizer and adjust the vulcanizer cover.

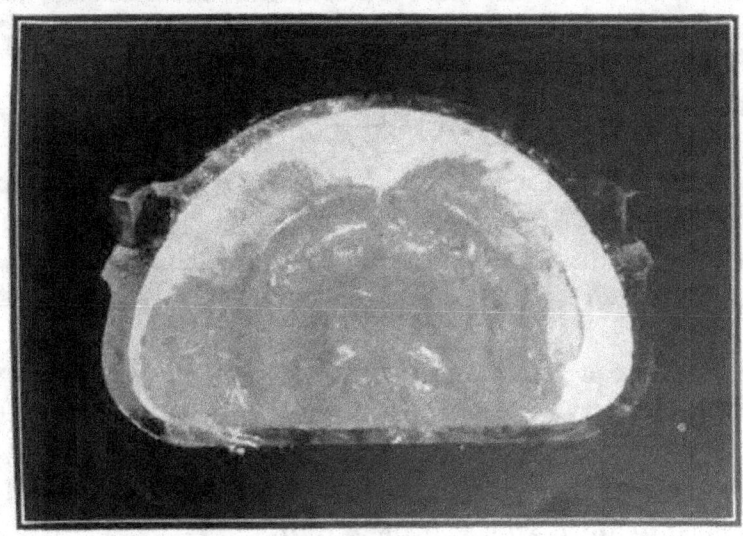

FIGURE 49.

c. Open the blow-off valve.

d. Light the burner under the pot and adjust it until the blue flame just covers the bottom of the vulcanizer. Never allow it to reach up the sides.

e. Set the gas regulator to 320°, or according to vulcanizing directions.

f. Allow all air to escape and when steam begins to be expelled, close the blow-off valve, using a wrench.

g. Set the time clock to shut off the gas at the required interval.

h. Vulcanize for 1½ hours from the time the blow-off valve is closed. Allow 35 minutes to reach 320°. Maintain this temperature for 55 minutes.

i. The time regulator will shut off the supply of gas as regulated.

j. Allow vulcanizer to cool for 15 minutes, then open blow-off valve until steam begins to escape.

k. After all steam has escaped, remove the vulcanizer cover.

l. Remove flask from vulcanizer and allow to cool for 15 minutes. Then place it in cold water until thoroughly chilled.

48. Cleansing and polishing dentures.—*a.* Remove the flask cover.

b. Using a plaster knife, remove the plaster from around the edges of the upper part of the flask until the teeth are exposed, as well as the buccal and labial surfaces of the denture.

c. With a knife inserted between the upper and lower portions of the flask, carefully open it without applying too much pressure.

d. Carefully remove the denture from all surrounding plaster.

e. Wash all excess plaster from the denture with a stiff bristle brush while holding it under cold water.

f. With a sharp pointed knife peel away all the tinfoil or cellophane from the tissue surface of the denture.

g. Cut away all excess vulcanite from the rim of the denture, being careful not to mar the peripheral border.

h. Partial dentures are removed in the same manner, only more care must be taken in their removal as they are easier to distort or fracture.

i. Using either a half-round vulcanite file or an abrasive wheel mounted on the lathe, remove all excess vulcanite from around the edge of the denture.

j. In partial dentures, use a rat tail vulcanite file around the cervical edges to bring it to the proper limits.

k. Remove all roughness from labial, buccal, palatal, and lingual surfaces of dentures by using a vulcanite scraper.

l. Carefully smooth the denture with sandpaper. In using sandpaper it is easy to take away too much vulcanite, thus exposing some dark rubber on the labial surface or making the denture too thin. It is also possible to harm the denture permanently by generating too much heat in this polishing process.

m. Carefully trim the vulcanite about the necks of the teeth on the buccal, labial, and lingual surfaces with sharp vulcanite trimmers. A sharp trimmer *must* always be used in this procedure to avoid undue pressure and to give a polished finish to the vulcanite.

n. All the steps previously described are preliminary to putting the final polish on the denture. It is necessary to obtain this high polish for the health and comfort of the patient. Vulcanite dentures are more or less porous and have a tendency to absorb saliva and accumulate food particles. High polish will reduce this porosity. Make a puttylike mix of fine pumice and water and, with a brush wheel rotating toward the operator, proceed to polish the denture. It should be held firmly in the hands, rocking it in a semicircular motion so that grooves will not be cut into the vulcanite. Always

DENTAL TECHNICIANS

keep the surface of the denture wet with pumice and use gentle pressure. Too much pressure will warp and burn the denture.

o. Repeat this process using a linen rag wheel with pumice in place of the brush wheel.

p. Mount large or small felt cones to the chuck of the lathe and polish all areas inaccessible with the rag wheel.

q. Make a mixture of chalk and water and with a soft flannel wheel continue to polish all surfaces of the denture.

r. Wash with water and check to make sure that all scratches have been removed. Then with a soft flannel wheel apply powdered oxide of tin for the final polish.

Section VII

ACRYLIC RESIN DENTURES

	Paragraph
General	49
Procedure	50

49. General.—The acrylic resins are used by the dental profession in order to have a denture material with better esthetic qualities than vulcanite and, at the same time, without sacrificing strength and durability. A great many synthetic materials have been developed and marketed from time to time, but the acrylic resins seem to be the best so far developed. There are various acrylic resins on the market and the procedure may vary slightly according to the material, but the basic technique is very much the same.

50. Procedure.—*a.* Wax up as if the denture were to be made of vulcanite, except that the wax should be a little fuller in the interproximal spaces to allow for tinfoiling.

b. Invest the case in the lower portion of the flask as for a vulcanite denture.

c. The cast is now ready for tinfoiling. This is a most important procedure in the construction of acrylic resin dentures as any error in this step will result in the final denture being weakened and spotted. It is necessary to have all surfaces *covered completely* with tinfoil. For the upper cast cut four pieces of tinfoil, one piece to fit the palate, two to fit the buccal surfaces, and one to fit the labial surface of the denture. Additional tinfoil is then cut to cover the plaster in the flask. The tinfoil for the lower case is the same with the exception of the part that will cover the lingual surfaces and the tongue spaces. This should be cut square and then rounded in front.

d. Cut the palatal piece of tinfoil into two triangular pieces. With a small piece of cotton, burnish the tinfoil on the wax of the palatal surface of the upper denture and overlap these two pieces in the center of the palate about ¼ inch. Extend the tinfoil to about ⅛ inch below the incisal and occlusal surfaces of the teeth.

e. Cut little V-shaped grooves in the tinfoil, covering the teeth on the labial, lingual, and buccal surfaces so it may be adapted into the interproximal spaces between the teeth.

f. Remove one side of the palatal tinfoil and apply glue to the overlapping margin and replace on the waxed case.

g. Adapt the labial and buccal pieces of tinfoil to the waxed surfaces from about ⅛ inch below the incisal and occlusal surfaces of the teeth. Use the separate pieces of tinfoil to cover the plaster surface. Seal the overlapping margins with glue (fig. 50).

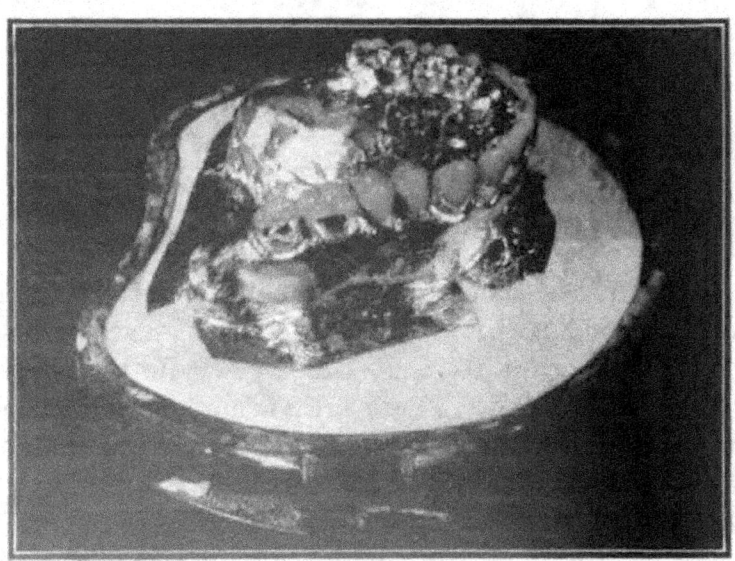

FIGURE 50.

h. In lower cases adapt a piece of tinfoil to cover the tongue space.

i. The remainder of the flasking procedure is identical to that used in vulcanite.

j. Boil out the wax in the same manner as previously described, washing the cast with chloroform followed by acetone. Make sure all acetone has evaporated before proceeding to pack the case.

k. In acrylic resin dentures it is necessary to tinfoil the cast. This is done after the case has been flasked and separated.

l. Acrylic resins usually come in two types. One type is the cake, and the other is the powder and liquid. The last mentioned is preferable and will be the one described. Have a clean sheet of paper about 8 inches square on the bench. Place the powder cup in which the material comes in the center of the sheet of paper and pour the powder the cup until it overflows. Scrape off all excess powder with a straightedge until the powder is level with the rim of the cup. Do not pack the material or jar it into the cup. Pour the powder so measured into any porcelain vessel such as a coffee cup. Measure out about 8 cc of the liquid and add to the powder in the cup. Immediately begin mixing vigorously with a clean, stiff, stainless steel spatula. Continue this mixing until the material begins to be homogeneous and loses most of its stickiness. This should take about 1 minute. Then roll the mixed material between the palms of the hands from 5 to 10 seconds. The hands should be clean and dry. For repairs, or if it is desired to make smaller or larger mixes than by the measuring cup, different quantities in correct proportions should be used.

m. The case is then ready to be packed. This should be done as quickly as possible after mixing. When first mixed, the material is very soft and easy to pack, but upon standing it becomes stiffer and requires more pressure to close the flask. The flasking should be done soon after boiling out so that the flask will be warm but not hot. A good temperature is 100° to 125° F. Roll between the hands a piece of the material about the size of a lead pencil and sufficiently long to cover the teeth. Pack this well down against the teeth, making sure that no air is inclosed. Next roll up another piece about the thickness of the little finger and long enough to go around the arch. Immediately press this to place with the fingers. In upper cases it is necessary to put a sheet of the material over the palate.

n. The flask may be trial-separated by placing a strip of moist cellophane over the material in the flask before closing. Close as quickly as possible in any convenient press. Do not apply any extra heat to the flask to facilitate closing as this will only hasten the setting of the material. The flask is then reopened and material either added or cut away as necessary. It is now ready for curing.

o. The case may be cured in a vulcanizer or in boiling water. Either way gives good results. In the vulcanizer, any curing temperature from 212° to 320° F. and a minimum time of 1 hour may be used. Cooling after curing is done in the same manner as for vulcanite.

p. The simplest manner in which to cure the denture is to place the case and the flask in a pan of cold water. This water is then brought to a boil and allowed to boil for about 40 minutes. The case is then allowed to cool very gradually (preferably overnight) before opening. The case is opened, the denture removed and polished in the same manner as previously described.

Section VIII

DENTURE REPAIR

	Paragraph
Simple repair	51
Loose or broken teeth	52
Teeth added	53
Loose clasp	54
Refacing	55
Rebasing	56
Duplicating denture	57
Repairing acrylic resin dentures	58

51. Simple repair.—*a.* Bring the fractured edges of the denture into apposition and seal them together with a little sticky wax. Pieces of stiff wire are laid over the fractured denture at right angles to the line of fracture and waxed in place. This gives the denture additional support.

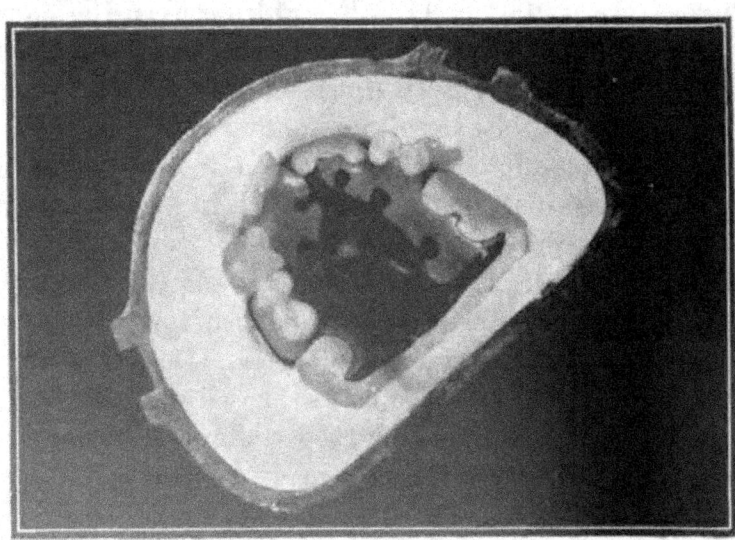

Figure 51.

b. Lubricate the tissue surface of the denture with petrolatum.

c. Place boxing wax around that part of the periphery of the denture that makes contact with the natural teeth.

d. Make a plaster mix and pour a matrix or cast of the denture as described in pouring impressions.

e. When the plaster has set, remove the denture parts and with abrasive chucks and vulcanite burs grind away a large portion of the palate on each side of the fracture. Also remove about 2 millimeters of vulcanite from the periphery of the denture over those areas containing artificial teeth. The margins of the palatal area are then dovetailed as shown.

f. Replace the fractured parts on the cast, fill in the missing parts of the vulcanite with wax, making this wax a little thicker than the original vulcanite. This will allow for the finishing and polishing of the denture (fig. 51).

g. Pour the lower and upper portions of the flask as done in a new case.

h. After the plaster has set, the wax is eliminated and the flask carefully opened. The denture will be contained in the upper half of the flask.

i. With a vulcanite bur remove about ½ millimeter of vulcanite from the entire tissue surface of the denture. The surface is roughened (fig. 52).

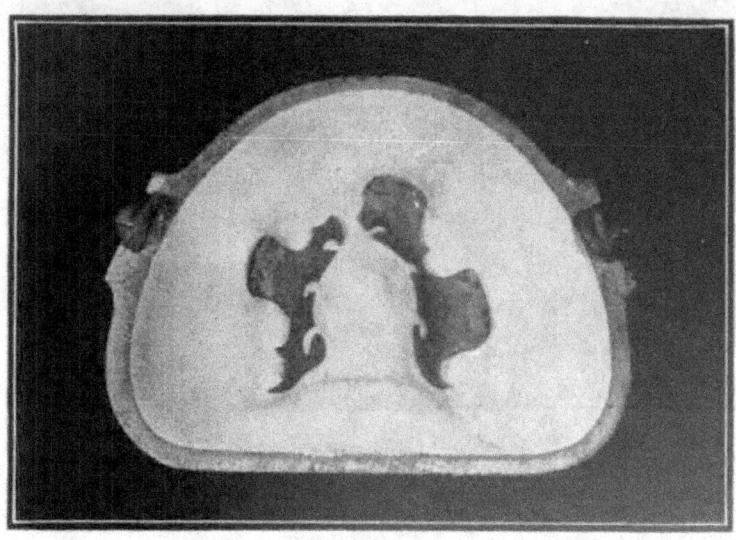

FIGURE 52.

j. Proceed to pack the case as usual and then place a piece of wet cellophane over the case before the final closing.

k. The case is then vulcanized and finished as previously described.

52. Loose or broken teeth.—*a.* When the original tooth has become loosened and can be replaced, it is only necessary to make certain it fits in its exact position as marked on the vulcanite. Then cut a dovetail in the lingual or palatal surface of the vulcanite adjacent to the tooth, replace the tooth in its original position, and secure it by wax. The case is then carried forward as in the simple repair.

b. When the tooth has been broken or lost and a new tooth is necessary but the denture base at the site of the tooth is intact, it is necessary for the dental officer to supply the technician with a wax bite indicating the relationship of the teeth of the opposing jaws. Proceed as in simple repair until matrix is poured. Fit the teeth of the denture into the depressions on the bite, and seal it to the denture. Fill the depressions left in the bite by the teeth of the opposing jaw with plaster. The matrix of the denture and the poured bite are then mounted on an articulator, after which the bite is removed. Place the new tooth in the correct position, as governed by the adjacent and opposing teeth. Do not grind away any of the vulcanite found around the neck of the tooth, but do all necessary grinding on the tooth itself. Wax into position and proceed as in simple repair.

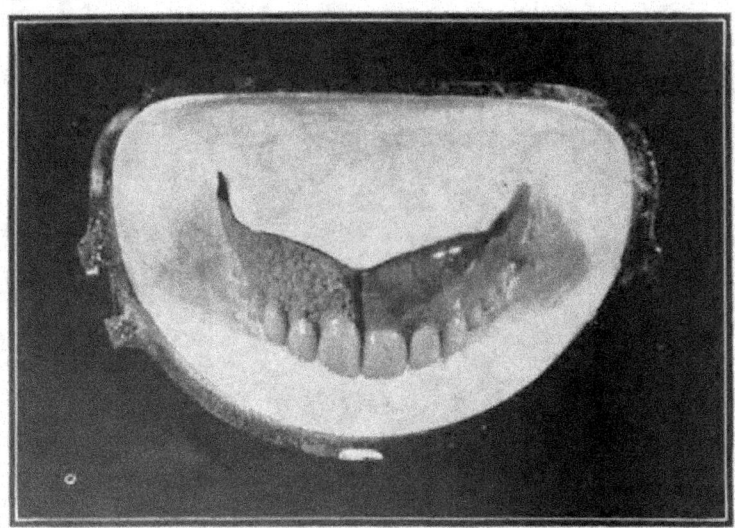

FIGURE 53.

53. Teeth added.—Often a tooth is extracted requiring the addition of an artificial tooth to a partial denture. The technician receives the impression of the mouth that has been taken with the denture in place. If the impression has been taken in plaster, it must be painted with a separating media. A wax rim is placed around the periphery of the denture and the cast is poured. The bite is placed in its correct position on the denture and waxed in place and poured. The denture, cast, and bite are then mounted on an articulator. The bite is removed and the additional teeth are added to the denture, as described above, and the process followed as in a simple repair.

54. Loose clasp.—The dental officer has taken an impression of the clasped tooth with the clasp and denture in position. The impression is poured as directed for adding teeth to a partial denture. The vulcanite is cut out from around the tailpiece of the clasp, and this area filled with wax. The case is then carried to completion as previously described.

55. Refacing.—Lubricate the inner surface of the denture and with plaster, forming a matrix. Allow to set. Cut away the labial and buccal vulcanite to about one-half of its original thickness, making certain the rubber is removed from around the necks of the teeth. Honeycomb the remaining gum rubber to roughen it. Wax the labial and buccal surfaces of the denture. Flask the case by filling the lower part of the flask with fairly stiff plaster and setting the denture into this plaster with the teeth down. Make sure that the teeth are at least ¼ inch from the bottom of the flask, and that all the waxed parts are exposed. Smooth the plaster around the teeth and over the rear of the denture. The upper part of the flask is poured after lubricating and the case is continued as in simple repairs (fig. 53).

56. **Rebasing.**—Often the gums will shrink or pull away from the denture after it has been worn for some time. This causes the denture to become loose and irritating to the patient. If the denture is in good condition otherwise, it may be repaired by adding a new base or foundation of vulcanite. The technician receives the denture, to the base of which has been added a sufficient amount of material to correct the deficiency in the mouth of the patient. This material is usually modeling compound, but it may be plaster or both. A strip of boxing wax is placed around the periphery of the denture and the cast is poured as described. The case is then flasked the same as if it were a new denture. After the two parts of the flask have been separated, the impression material is removed. The tissue surface of the denture is roughened by vulcanite burs and stones to facilitate the addition of the new vulcanite. Sufficient vulcanite should be removed to allow for about 1 millimeter of new rubber. The case is packed with strips of base rubber, the flask is closed and the case carried to completion as previously described.

57. **Duplicating denture.**—Frequently it is necessary to replace the entire denture base with new material. The technique as given here does not require the case to be mounted on an articulator. Proceed as in any simple repair until the matrix is poured. Make several deep grooves on the buccal and labial surfaces of the old denture. Lubricate the teeth and the buccal and labial surfaces of the denture and matrix. Build a plaster index around the entire outer surfaces of the denture and matrix, extending the plaster to about ¼ inch from the incisal and occlusal surfaces of the teeth. Before the plaster sets too hard, make a cut opposite each cuspid tooth. This weakens the plaster index which is carefully removed as soon as it is sufficiently hard. Lift the denture from the matrix and remove all the teeth from the denture by covering them with a layer

melted basewax and then passing the denture several times through a flame to soften the vulcanite. The teeth are arranged in their proper position as indicated on the plaster index, and are secured with sticky wax. A baseplate is constructed over the matrix and the plaster index containing the teeth is arranged around the matrix with the baseplate. Melted basewax is flowed into the spaces between the teeth and the baseplate. The sticky wax holding the teeth is removed as well as the index. The waxing is finished where necessary without disturbing the position of the teeth. Proceed with the flasking as described. It is sometimes necessary to use basewax instead of the baseplate to avoid displacing the teeth in the index.

58. Repairing acrylic resin dentures.—Bring the broken parts of the denture into apposition and wax them securely together. A cast is then poured as in the vulcanite case. The model is then removed and tinfoiled. Replace the denture on the model and rewax if necessary. Tinfoil the complete denture, holding it in place with a little thin glue. Do not tinfoil the wax portions. Flask as for a vulcanite repair. Boil out the wax, but do not use chloroform or acetone to clean the cast. Tinfoil the plaster in the upper half of the flask that will come in contact with the denture or the repair portions. A small mix of the powder and liquid is made, as previously described, and this material is packed in the repair portion and the flask closed. The denture is cured as for a full denture. If the case has undercuts so that the denture cannot be removed from the cast, it is necessary to tinfoil the denture before pouring the model.

Section IX

DENTAL CASTINGS

	Paragraph
General	59
Requirements	60
Methods	61
Procedure	62

59. General.—Many dental restorations, completely or in part, are made by carving a wax pattern and reproducing that wax pattern in gold by a process known as casting. Castings of gold alloys may be made with considerable accuracy for anything from the largest partial denture to the smallest inlay. However, this section takes up only the construction of the smaller pieces. The fundamental procedure is the same for the large castings as for the small, the technical differences which must be observed in large castings being brought out in section XIV.

60. Requirements.—There are many requirements in making a satisfactory casting. The wax pattern must be carefully prepared to fit the model or die, and the casting made from the wax pattern must approximate the size and shape of the wax pattern very closely. The metal used must have satisfactory properties for casting as well as for making it capable of withstanding the forces to which it will be subjected. Assuming the alloy to be of the desired composition it must then be cast properly to prevent imperfections in the final structure. After casting, the alloy must be cleaned, polished, and often heat-treated to produce the desired physical properties in the metal.

61. Methods.—*a.* The dentist sometimes carves the pattern for the inlay or crown in the mouth of the patient and furnishes the dental technician with the completed wax pattern. This is known as the direct method and is used extensively, especially on smaller castings.

b. However, the dentist often takes a compound impression of the tooth and a metal die is made from this. This is known as the indirect method. In this method the dental technician will be presented with the impression from which he must first make an amalgam die and then make a wax pattern on the amalgam die. The die is made by wrapping a sheet of thin wax around the impression of the tooth, imbedding the whole in a ring of plaster, and packing amalgam tightly into the mold thus formed to give a reproduction of the crown of the tooth together with a rootlike extension for handling in the subsequent steps. The procedure for constructing a die is taken up in greater detail in section X.

c. When large castings are made, a model of part or all of the jaw is poured in the actual casting investment and the wax pattern formed directly on this model. This procedure is taken up in section XIV.

62. Procedure.—The following are the steps for making a small casting, using a metal die:

a. The die is lubricated with a thin coating of cocoa butter. Petrolatum or light machine oil may be used but cocoa butter is not absorbed as readily by the wax and makes the later removal of the wax pattern easier.

b. Soften the wax in an open flame or in an oven or water bath until it is uniformly and thoroughly plastic.

c. Adapt the softened mass of wax to the die and press forcibly to place so that the wax will be closely conformed to the surface of the die.

d. Add melted wax with a spatula to make up for any deficiencies or correct any flaws in the wax mass.

e. Carefully carve the wax to the desired shape, reproducing the anatomical characteristics of the tooth.

f. Attach a short section of round wire (sprue) to the pattern and gently remove it from the die, using the sprue pin as a handle. The sprue pin is attached at its free end to a sprue base or crucible former which fits on the end of the casting ring and forms a depression in the investment for the melting of the gold during the casting process. While no set rule exists as to the placing of the sprue pin, it should be placed in a position to facilitate the flow of the molten gold into the mold. The following rules should be observed in placing the sprue:

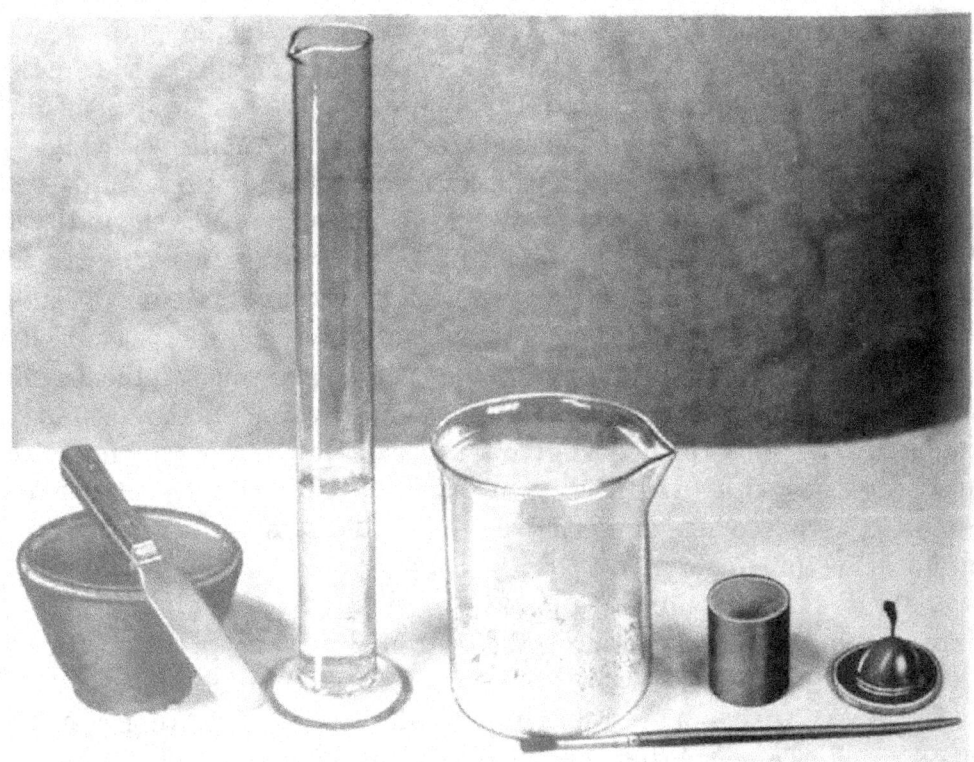

FIGURE 54.—Materials used in investing pattern for casting: Plaster bowl and spatula; correct amount of water (weighed or measured); correct amount of investment; casting ring containing an inner lining of asbestos; wax pattern fixed to crucible former; and camel's-hair brush.

(1) The sprue should not be attached to the **center of a broad, flat** surface.

(2) The sprue should not be attached so that **the molten metal will** strike directly against a fine margin.

(3) A minimum number of sprues should be used (**only one on small** castings).

Figure 54 shows the materials used in investing the wax pattern. The wax pattern affixed to a brass crucible former by a sprue pin is shown at the extreme right.

g. Wash the wax pattern thoroughly in cold water with a fine camel's-hair brush and a soap solution.

h. Mix the casting investment according to the manufacturer's directions, being careful to avoid incorporating air bubbles in the mix. Air bubbles can be avoided by mechanical spatulation, spatulating the mix for a considerable time, and vibrating the mix either by hand or on a mechanical vibrator for a few seconds after mixing.

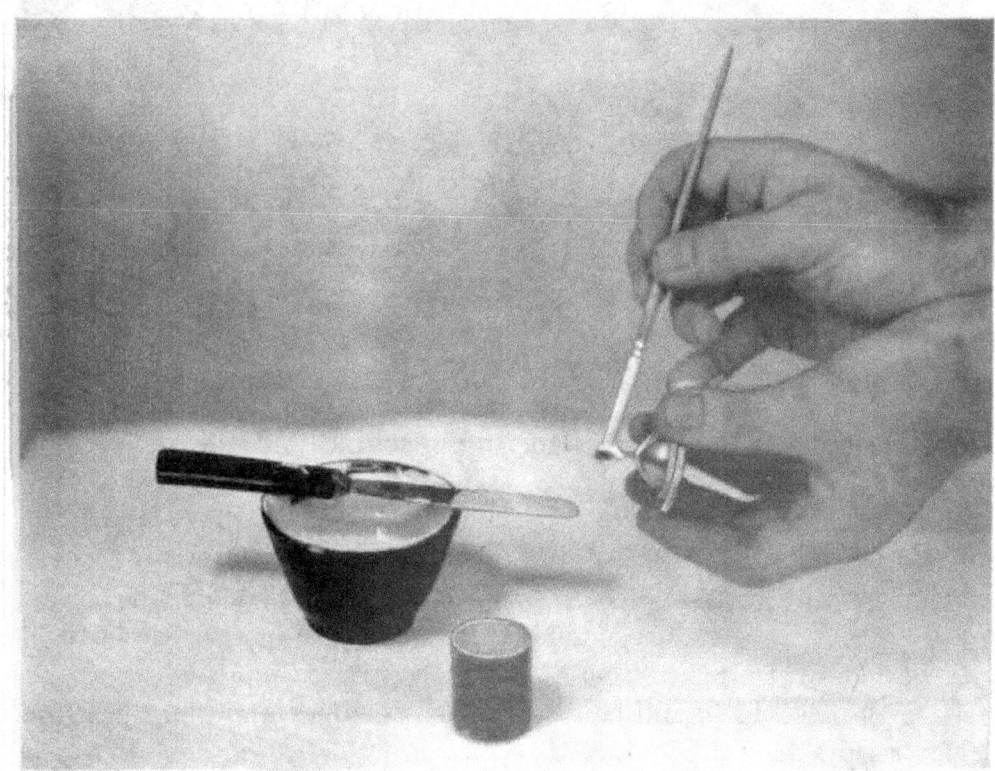

FIGURE 55.—Coating wax pattern with investment prior to placing it in ring.

i. Carefully paint some of the investment on the wax pattern with a camel's-hair brush, flowing a small amount of investment ahead of the brush to avoid trapping air bubbles on the surface of the pattern (fig. 55).

j. After coating the pattern for the first time, blow off as much of the investment as possible, thus exposing any trapped air bubbles. Then coat the pattern again, being careful to flow the investment ahead of the brush so as not to incorporate air bubbles.

k. Fill the casting ring with the investment and carefully set the investment-covered pattern in the ring (fig. 56).

l. After the investment sets, remove the sprue former and sprue, and place the ring in an oven to eliminate the wax. The ring is ready for casting when a cherry-red glow can be seen down the sprue hole.

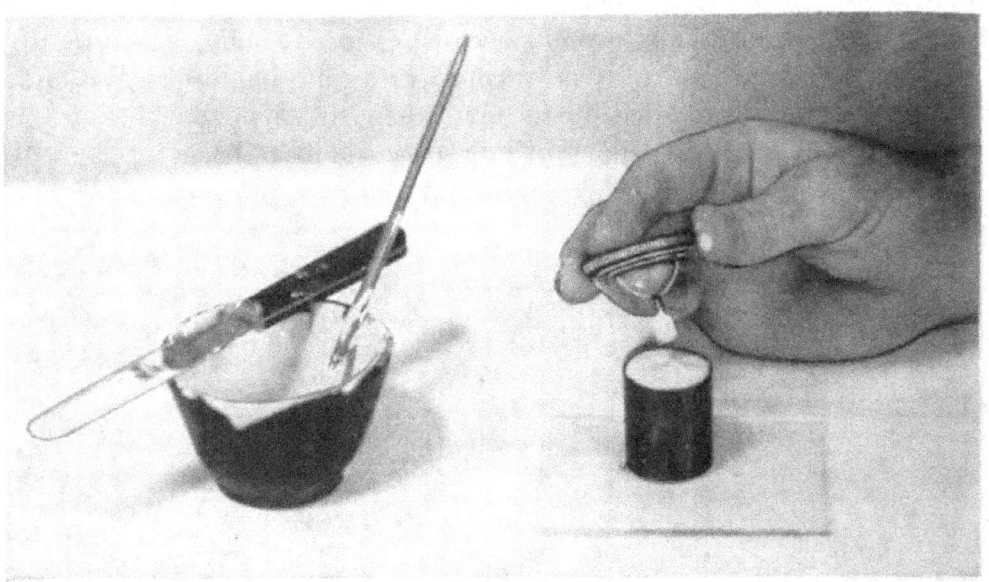

FIGURE 56.—Immersing coated pattern into investment-filled casting ring.

m. The ring is placed in a casting machine and the gold alloy melted with a blowtorch flame. The correct temperature of the molten gold is determined by experience in observing the color of the gold which should be heated to light yellow (almost white) heat. Enough gold alloy must be used to fill competely the mold and sprue and leave an excess in the crucible; this excess is known as the button. The period of time between taking the ring from the oven and making the casting should be as short as possible; less than 1 minute if best results are to be obtained.

n. After casting, the metal is removed from the investment and cleaned with a brush. The gold is then pickled by boiling in a concentrated solution (30 to 40 percent) of sulfuric or hydrochloric acid. The pickling removes oxides and other debris in preparation for finishing.

SECTION X

CAST CROWNS

	Paragraph
General	63
Obtaining model	64
Investing and casting	65

63. General.—Three-quarter crowns and full crowns are generally used as attachments for fixed bridges. The three-quarter crown has the advantage over the full gold crown in that it does not show as much gold. The three-quarter crown is retained on the tooth by two parallel grooves which are cut in the mesial and distal surfaces

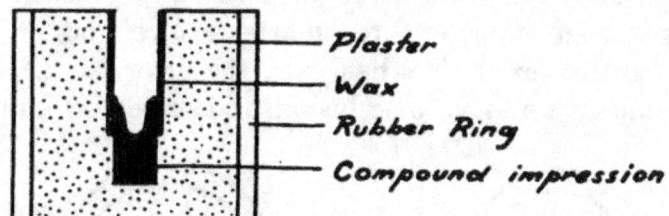

FIGURE 57.—Cross section diagram of tooth impression set in ring of plaster ready to receive die amalgam.

of the tooth. In addition to these grooves, often a groove is cut on the incisal edge or holes for pins are placed on either the incisal edge or lingual surface for added stability and retention.

64. Obtaining model.—*a.* For full or partial crowns an impression is taken of the tooth and a metal die or model is made usually of amalgam as was mentioned in section IX. As is described in that section, the dentist takes an impression of the tooth with compound in the copper band. For a crown, additional impressions are taken in plaster or other materials of the surrounding teeth and of the opposing teeth. The die or model of the tooth to be crowned is made first by packing amalgam into the impression which has been boxed by wrapping wax or gummed paper around the brass band and sinking it in a ring of plaster (fig. 57).

b. An amalgam model is made by mixing in a mortar and pestle seven parts of amalgam alloy and five parts of mercury by weight, and triturating for 3 minutes. This amalgam is worked in the palm of the hand for 2 or 3 minutes until it has been thoroughly mixed. Then, using a small amalgam plugger, it is packed into the impression of the tooth, a small amount at a time. The mold is filled even with the plaster so that a rootlike extension is formed on the amalgam die or model of the tooth. After the amalgam has set, the plaster is broken away and the band removed after immersing in hot water. The rootlike part of the die is trimmed with stones.

c. This die is now put into place in the plaster impression of the jaw and a stone model is poured with the amalgam die in place. This will give a stone model of the jaw or section of the jaw, with the amalgam die in place in the model. With a stone model of the upper poured and both models mounted on a small crown and bridge articu-

TM 8-225
64-66 MEDICAL DEPARTMENT

lator, the wax pattern on the die then can be carved. The wax pattern is constructed as described in section IX. However, it must be carved to articulate properly with the opposing model.

65. Investing and casting.—The technique for investing and casting the gold crown, whether three-quarter or full, is the same as described in section IX. The sprue pin is usually placed on the disto-incisal edge in an anterior three-quarter crown and on a lingual cusp for a posterior crown. When cast, the crown is fitted on the die, trimmed and adjusted as to occlusion, and smoothed and polished.

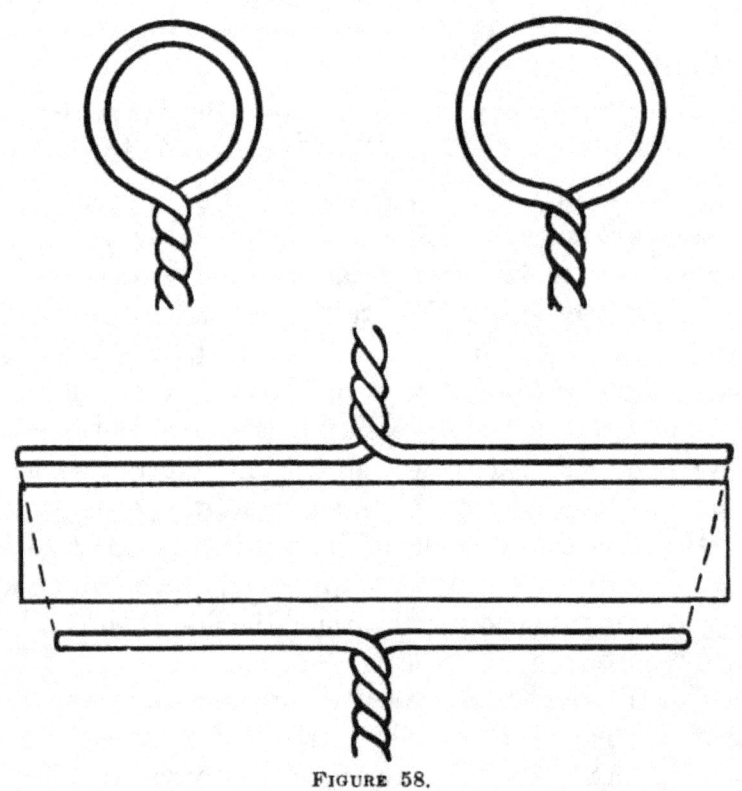

FIGURE 58.

SECTION XI

CAST OCCLUSAL GOLD CROWN

	Paragraph
General	66
Procedure	67

66. General.—The cast occlusal gold crown is another type of full crown frequently used. In this technique a gold band is adapted around a model of the tooth and only the occlusal is cast. Due to the requirements of esthetics, it is employed for restoring posterior teeth only. The primary requirement in the construction of the cast gold crown is an accurate fit at the gingival line. One of the most serious faults of the full gold crown is the frequent occurrence of caries under the band. This can nearly always be traced to the failure in securing close adaptation of the band to the tooth at the margin. In order to obtain this adaptation the dental officer will take two measurements with a dentimeter of the prepared tooth stump. The first is taken around the neck of the tooth at the gum line and the second measurement is taken in a similar manner at a point about one-third the length of the stump from the occlusal surface. These measurements are taken by looping a piece of wire around the tooth at each one of the points mentioned above, and tightening the wire by twisting the ends. The two loops thus formed are removed from the tooth and cut. When they are straightened out they will give the exact circumference of the crown of the tooth at each one of these points (fig. 58).

67. Procedure.—*a.* The measurement wires are cut and straightened out.

b. A piece of 22-carat, 30-gage gold plate is cut slightly wider than the length of the tooth stump. It is cut to a length that is ½ millimeter longer than that of the longer measurement wire to allow for beveling. The shorter wire is placed along the lower edge of the gold plate, equidistant from the ends and its length marked on the gold with a pointed instrument. This measurement is also increased ½ millimeter to allow for beveling. It is seen that since one of the measurement wires is shorter than the other, the gold plate will not be cut as a rectangle, but the ends will converge slightly toward the shorter wire. Cut the band along these guide lines, as illustrated in figure 58.

c. Bevel the gold band at each end at an angle of 45°. using a flat file. The file is passed over the band in only one direction. The bevel is placed on the opposite side at the other end of the band so that the two beveled surfaces will overlap when the band is curved.

d. The best method of uniting the ends of the band is autogenous soldering or sweating. This can only be done when pieces of gold of the same carat are to be united. By this means the parts are melted or welded together without using solder. When this method is used there is no danger of the joint becoming disunited in subsequent solderings. The beveled ends of the band are bent around and under each other until the ends overlap. These ends are then pulled back and allowed to spring together upon each other, thus pressing together by the elasticity of the metal. This exact contact of the ends is necessary in autogenous soldering. The joint is fluxed with a saturated solution of borax, and the band is placed on a piece of charcoal with the lapped edges up. Using a blowpipe, start with a small brush flame, continue to apply heat until the band is brought to a cherry red. When the gold begins to glisten the surfaces are nearly ready to fuse. Remove the flame immediately after the parts are united. The band is returned to the dental officer, who trims and fits it to the gum line of the tooth.

e. The united band is then placed upon a flat surface and the occlusal edge is filed until it is in flat contact with the file. When the band is in place on the tooth stump, the occlusal edge should be the exact height of the occlusal surface of the preparation.

f. In constructing a gold crown for a pulpless tooth, a piece of 22-carat, 30-gage gold plate of a size large enough to cover the occlusal end of the band is selected. One side is coated with a solution of borax. The gold band is then placed on the gold plate and they are held in a bunsen burner with a pair of tweezers until the band is sweated to the gold plate. The excess gold of the plate is cut away so that the margins are smooth and the crown boxlike. This step is only used for pulpless teeth. The technique for vital teeth will be taken up later.

g. A wax bite and a plaster impression are now taken by the dental officer.

h. Select a porcelain tooth having a well-developed occlusal anatomy and of a width which will fill the space formerly occupied by the natural tooth. The occlusal surface of this tooth is covered with a coating of oil and then forced into a small block of modeling compound, the surface of which has been softened. The compound is chilled and the porcelain tooth removed, leaving an impression of its occlusal surface in the compound. The surface of the impression is covered with a thin coat of oil and softened inlay wax is forced into the impression. The wax is chilled and trimmed flat and level with the block of modeling compound. It is then removed from the block. The gold coping is placed on the cast and the wax occlusal form is placed in position on the coping. The wax is then carved and adjusted where necessary to conform to the occlusion of the opposing teeth. Inlay wax is added to the approximal, lingual, and buccal surfaces of the gold coping and carved until the proper contour of the tooth is obtained. About 1 millimeter of gold band is left exposed at the gum margin.

i. Attach the sprue at one corner of the crown, invest, and cast as described under the three-quarter crown.

j. Twenty-two-carat gold solder is fused over the exposed band with the blowpipe to perfect the contour around the gingival margin of the crown. The crown is cleaned in acid and polished.

k. When the cast gold crown is used on a vital tooth, no attempt is made to place a gold floor on the band, due to the irregular border at the occlusal surface, which is usually unavoidable in vital teeth. After the gold band has been accurately fitted at the gingival margin, the occlusal surface of the band is reduced with stones to the same height as the tooth stump. An impression and bite is then taken with the modeling compound, and the gold band is placed in the modeling compound impression. From this bite impression articulated stone casts are prepared. Wax cusps are added and carved to occlusal adaptation and the crown is then cast and finished, as described.

Section XII

FIXED BRIDGE

	Paragraph
General	68
Models	69
Construction of bridge	70
Other methods	71

68. General.—The fixed bridge consists of artificial teeth supported by crowns or inlays affixed to natural teeth adjoining the space. Because the artificial teeth so placed are rigidly fastened to each other and also fastened to crowns or inlays at both ends, this restoration is called a bridge. The crowns or inlays which support the appliance are called *abutments* and the natural teeth which receive these restorations are called *abutment teeth*. Crown construction and dental casting have been discussed in previous sections. The first step in constructing a bridge is the construction of crowns or inlays for the natural teeth adjoining the space.

69. Models.—After the construction of the crowns (or other castings) which are to hold the bridge, the dentist takes an impression of the mouth with the crowns in place. This impression containing the abutment crowns is poured in an investment material so that the model so formed may be used for casting or soldering. Also an impression of the opposing teeth is taken and a bite to articulate the two models thus obtained. The dental technician therefore starts a bridge from an investment model which contains the abutment crowns and a model of plaster or stone of the opposing teeth. These models are mounted on a crown and bridge articulator. The dental surgeon also furnishes the technician with the shade of the porcelain teeth desired.

70. Construction of bridge.—*a.* The first step consists of selecting the type of porcelain bridge tooth which will be used. Many types of porcelain tooth replacements for use on fixed bridgework are manufactured. The most commonly used are the Steele's type facing. This consists of a facing of porcelain which slides on a key affixed to a metal backing. The porcelain has a groove molded in the back which accurately fits the key and so retains the facing (fig. 59). Other types of porcelain facings include the long-pin facing and the short-pin facing. These are facings which are retained by means of two metal pins baked into the back of the porcelain. The long-pin facings are used in constructing cast gold bridges and the short-pin facings are used in constructing the old solder-type bridge. In addition to facings, there are bridge pontics. These are porcelain members which are so constructed that they furnish a complete porcelain contact with the soft tissue, and the gold portion of the bridge

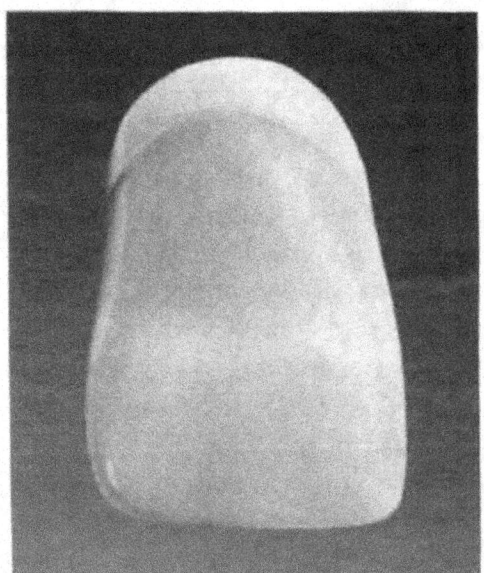 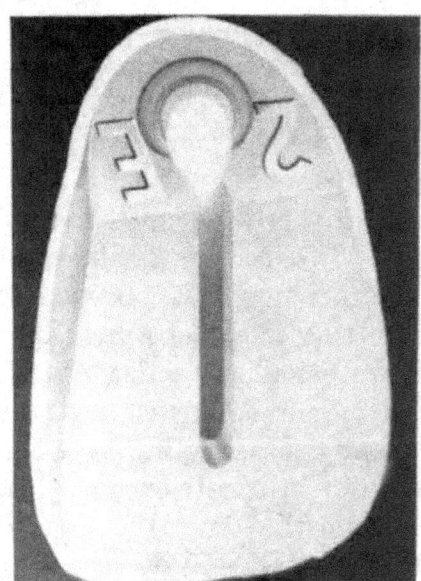

FIGURE 59.—Steele's facing showing slot which is molded in back to receive metal key of backing.

will not touch the gum tissue at all. These are the best type of bridge teeth from all standpoints if the length of the abutment teeth and other mechanical factors permit their use. However, the most commonly used type is the Steele facing which is on the supply table.

b. The next step consists of grinding and fitting the porcelain pontics or facings. The proper facings are selected by placing some soft wax on the model in the space and trying in various sizes and molds of teeth until the best possible selection is obtained. The best size facing for a case is one which is exactly the right width but which is somewhat longer than the space because it must be ground to fit the ridge. If the facings fit the case very well, little grinding is needed. The facings, however, must accurately fit the ridge and this fit is accomplished by grinding. The incisal or occlusal edge of the facing should be ground very little if at all (fig. 60).

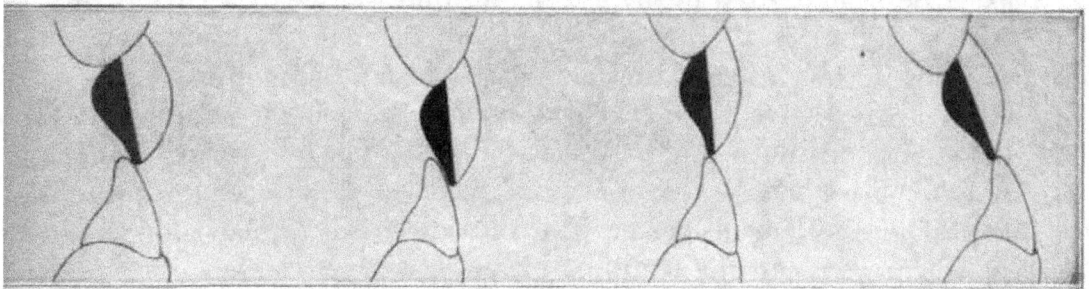

NOTE.—Black portion represents finished gold casting and shows proper relation of gold portion to facing. Notice how porcelain facing is protected in each case by slight extension of gold.

FIGURE 60.—Cross section diagrams of facings ground to fit ridge.

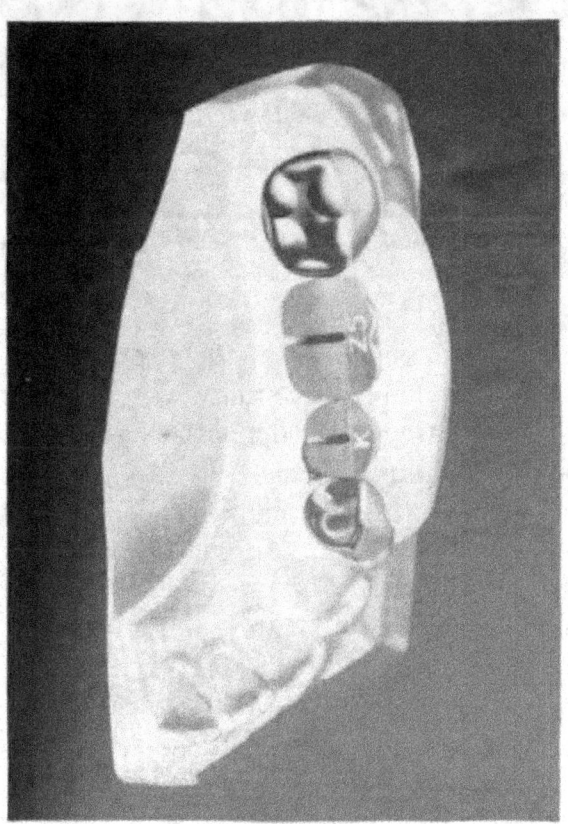

NOTE.—In this case porcelain pontics are used but template is used in same manner with facings.

FIGURE 61.—Plaster template in place on model.

c. A metal backing is selected to fit the porcelain facings. The backing should extend slightly above the incisal or occlusal edge of the facing to protect the facing from breakage. The backing is then ground flush with the facing on all sides except the incisal; here it is beveled toward the porcelain so that a hair line of backing extends above the porcelain to take the biting stress (fig. 60).

d. The facings with the backings in place are now arranged in the exact position desired in the finished bridge and fixed in this position with sticky wax. The outside surface of the model is lubricated with vaseline in the region of the facings and a small amount of plaster is poured over the facial side of the facings and on the surface of the model around the facings. When this little plaster section hardens, it is removed and serves as a guide which may be used to establish the facings in their proper position during the subsequent steps. This plaster piece is called a template (fig. 61).

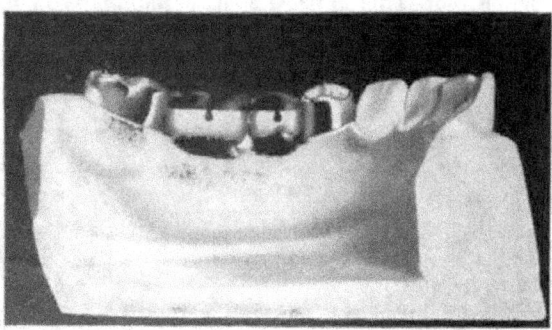

Note.—When facings are used instead of pontics, case is handled in same manner.
Figure 62.—Pontics sticky-waxed to model prior to adding casting wax to form wax pattern.

e. The facings are assembled in the proper position by means of the template and then affixed by sticky wax in that position (fig. 62). Melted inlay wax is then placed on the backings and in such bulk as to form a sizable reinforcement and to restore the shape of the teeth that the facings represent. This wax is then carved to the desired shape, reproducing the anatomy of the lingual or tongue side of the facing. In posterior teeth this wax restoration must be made to occlude with the opposing teeth for this will be the shape of the finished bridge.

f. This wax pattern of the gold portion of the pontics is then removed from the model with the porcelain facings in place. One or more sprues are added and the porcelain facings are slipped off the backings (fig. 63). The whole is invested and cast. Care must be taken not to heat the case too hot in the burning-out process as the metal backings are invested and it is not desired to melt or distort them.

g. After casting, the backings usually will be satisfactorily united to the casting in the process. Where any flaws exist between the backing and the casting proper they must be corrected by solder.

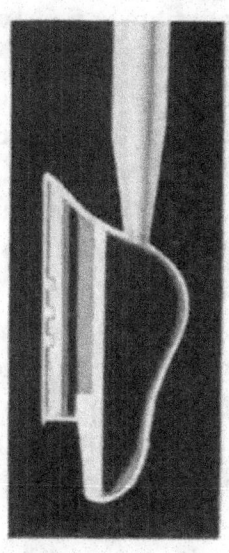 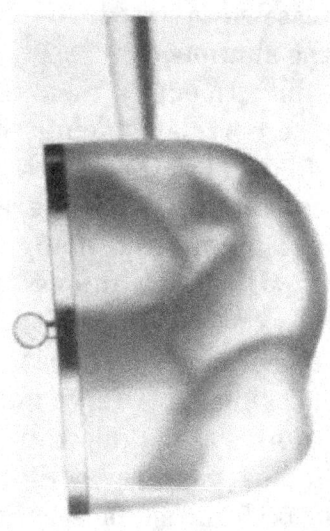

Note.—Notice that sprues are placed so that the molten gold will not strike directly against metal backings when casting.

Figure 63.—Wax patterns and attached backings of single-tooth bridges (one anterior and one posterior) sprued and ready for casting.

h. After cleaning and shaping the casting, the porcelain facings are placed on it and the whole assembled on the model with the aid of the plaster template (fig. 64).

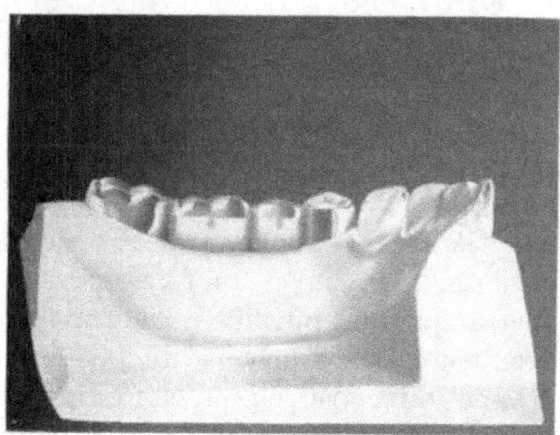

Note.—Metal portion of bridge will now be sticky-waxed to abutment crowns, pontics (or facings) removed, investment material placed in space to affix casting to model, and casting then soldered to abutments.

Figure 64.—Whole bridge assembled prior to soldering.

i. The bridge casting is sticky-waxed in place, the template removed, and the facings slipped out, leaving the metal part of the bridge sticky-waxed to the model in the proper position.

j. After soaking the model, investment material is mixed and placed on the model and over the facing part of the casting, firmly joining the casting to the model to which the abutments are affixed.

k. With the case so invested, the bridge portion is firmly soldered at each end to the abutments.

l. All of the investment is then removed. The case, pickled and polished, with the porcelain facings is now ready for delivery to the dental surgeon for trial in the mouth.

71. Other methods.—There are numerous variations of the above-described technique and many other techniques of constructing bridges. Most of these techniques are satisfactory, but the above procedure will give excellent results and is a fairly simple and rapid system. It may be mentioned that a common procedure consists of uniting all the backings by a large quantity of gold solder and adding enough solder to give the whole thing bulk so that no casting is necessary. This method, however, will only do where anterior teeth are replaced as the occlusal surface cannot be constructed with it, and also it does not give as precise and fine a result as a cast bridge.

Section XIII

CLASPS AND BARS FOR PARTIAL DENTURES

	Paragraph
General	72
Wrought clasps	73
Occlusal rests	74
Heat treatment of gold	75
Crib clasps	76
Cast clasps	77
Lingual and palatal bars	78

72. General.—*a.* Clasps are simple, direct retainers applied to two or more opposite, sloping, or convex surfaces of remaining natural teeth, which are chosen for that purpose during the designing of the denture. For convenience clasps may be divided into three classes, one-arm, two-arm, and three-arm clasps, according to the number of arms which are applied to the surfaces of the tooth. These may be either wrought or cast clasps. The former are constructed by bending a piece of gold clasp wire to conform to the tooth, and the latter are constructed by casting the clasps, using a special gold alloy. Both types have a definite place in dentistry and although there are many variations of both, this manual will deal only with those types are commonly used. In order to understand the construction of a clasp, no matter what type it may be, it is necessary to study the shape and contour of the crowns of the teeth so that these surfaces may be used to the best advantage. The fundamental reason behind

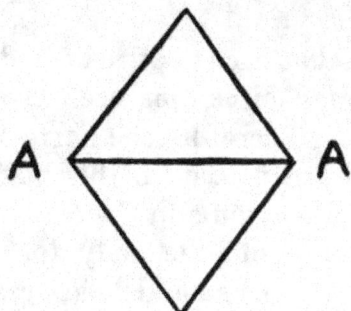

① Diagrammatic sketch illustrating line of greatest circumference of tooth.

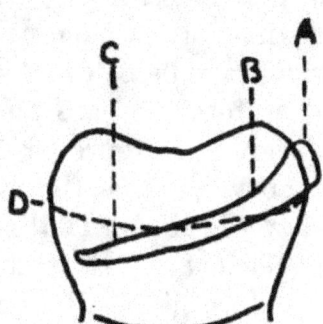

A. Body of clasp.　B. Shoulder of clasp.　C. Arm of clasp.　D. Line of greatest circumference on tooth.

② Arms of clasp below line of greatest circumference.

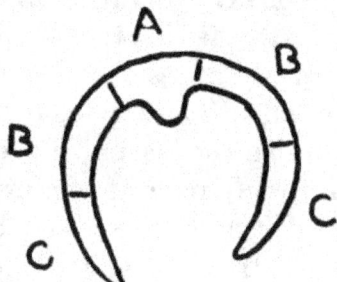

A. Body of clasp showing occlusal rest.　B. Shoulders of clasp.　C. Arms of clasp.

③ Sketch of clasp illustrating various parts.

FIGURE 65.

all clasps is to obtain the maximum amount of retention for the denture, and still allow it to be easily inserted and removed from the mouth. It must be understood that it is impractical to clasp some teeth due to their anatomical characteristics or position; therefore, it is essential that the dental officer take great care in the designing of the case. The three simple diagrams in figure 65 will clarify the fundamental mechanical theory which must be understood in order to construct efficient clasps.

b. Figure 65① shows that each tooth is divided into two separate parts by its line of greatest circumference. Nothing above this line can be used for retention. Therefore the parts of the clasp for which no retention is obtained are placed on this half of the tooth. This includes the body or rigid portion and the occlusal rest. The parts of the clasp that extend out from the body for a short distance are known as the shoulders. As the shoulders are relied upon for rigidity and not for retention, they should be placed either on the line of greatest circumference or just crossing it. Extending from these shoulders are the thin flexible arms from which the retention is derived. These arms must always be below the guideline and in the undercut of the tooth. Therefore they are placed below the line of greatest circumference, as shown in figure 65②. The body and occlusal rest of the clasps are above the line, the shoulders on or crossing the line, and the arms below the line. If this rule is followed, the clasp will give maximum efficiency. It is the duty of the dental officer to survey each case before giving it to the dental technician. marking on the cast the teeth to be clasped, the outline of the clasp and rest areas, and the outline of the entire denture. In a partial denture with two or more clasps, it is necessary to take into consideration the fact that while one clasp may be easily removed from the tooth, another clasp when attached to the denture may be in such a position as to make its removal impossible. Therefore, a mean vertical plane must be determined when the case is surveyed, which will coincide with the path along which the clasps will tend to seat themselves when attached to the denture. This is known as the *path of insertion.*

73. Wrought clasps.—Wrought clasps are constructed by bending a piece of either round or half-round gold clasp wire of the desired gage to conform to the tooth to be clasped. One of the most commonly used methods is to clasp a tooth adjoining a space caused by the extraction of one or more teeth. This allows sufficient room for the body of the clasp. However, it is frequently necessary to clasp a tooth which is in contact with the teeth on each side of it. As there is no room between the teeth to accommodate the body of the clasp, a different design must be used. However, the actual bending of the wire is done the same in each case. In the simple three-arm clasp, using a tooth adjoining a space, the following technique is followed:

a. Anneal the wire before any bending is attempted. This is done by holding it in an open flame until it assumes a cherry-red color. It is then plunged in cold water which removes the stiffness from the wire and makes it much easier to bend into shape. This annealing process should be repeated after each bending during the construction of the clasp.

b. Place one end of the wire on the lingual surface of the tooth where the outline of the clasp terminates, and note the point where the wire leaves the surface of the tooth. Grasp the wire with suit-

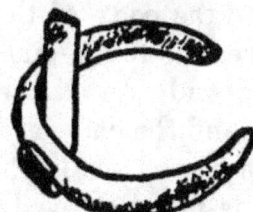

FIGURE 66.—Diagram of construction of occlusal rest.

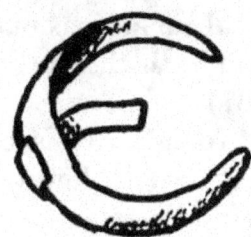

FIGURE 67.

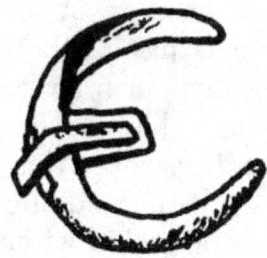

FIGURE 68.

able wire bending pliers and bend it slightly so that a greater length of the wire comes in contact with the tooth when tried on the model. It is then annealed and the point where it again leaves the tooth is noted and bent as before. This procedure is carried out until the clasp is conformed to the entire outline of the clasp on the model. As the buccal end of the clasp is approached, the length of wire to be used is judged and the remainder cut off with a pair of cutting pliers. The ends of the clasp are rounded with stones and burlew disks.

74. Occlusal rests.—*a.* In practically every partial denture case it is necessary to construct a third arm or occlusal rest as part of the clasp. This part will extend from the body of the clasp over the marginal ridge of the tooth and rest on a small section of the occlusal surface.

In this way the tooth can actually be made to bear most of the stresses of mastication instead of the tissue surfaces, and prevent the denture from settling down and forcing the clasp onto the gingival tissue around the neck of the tooth. Since the occlusal rest must bear quite a load it must be of sufficient strength to prevent breakage. A small piece of 36-gage pure gold plate is placed against the model at a point corresponding to the body of the clasp (fig. 66).

b. The clasp is placed over the tooth, and the end of the gold plate below the clasp is bent up and around the wire clasp, and secured with sticky wax. The lug and the clasp are removed from the model and soldered together with a very small piece of solder, making certain that the relationship is not destroyed. The clasp with the lug is then replaced on the model and the pure gold is burnished over the small part of the occlusal surface, as outlined on the model. The gold is trimmed to conform with the outline, leaving a small excess around the margins (fig. 67).

c. A short piece of half-round wire is bent to the shape of an L and laid over the rest as shown in figure 68. When soldered, this wire will reinforce the occlusal rest.

d. The clasp, lug, and wire are removed from the model and carefully invested in a small amount of investment material. The investment is allowed to come just to the margins of the lug. The investment is allowed to set and then gradually heated over an open flame until quite hot. Using a blowtorch, small pieces of either 18- or 20-carat gold solder are fused over this lug, further attaching it to the clasp and at the same time adding thickness to the lug so that it will have sufficient strength to withstand the stresses of mastication. The clasp with the occlusal rest is removed from the investment and polished. It is returned to the model and checked for accuracy. This procedure is repeated for all clasps requiring occlusal rests.

75. Heat treatment of gold.—As the repeated annealing of the gold clasp wire causes it to become soft and pliable, it is necessary to restore its hardness and elasticity by retempering after the work has been finished. To do this, the clasp is placed in an oven and heated to a temperature of 840° F., and held at that temperature for 10 minutes. It is then allowed to cool to 480° F. over a period of 30 minutes. If an oven is not available, heat in an open flame to cherry red and allow to cool in air.

76. Crib clasps.—*a.* The design of the clasps may be altered to suit the case. Frequently it is necessary to construct a clasp for a tooth which is in contact with the adjoining teeth. An example of this type of clasp is shown in figure 69.

b. In this type of attachment the body of the clasp is placed in the embrasure between the teeth instead of beside the distal or mesial surfaces. Preparation for this should be made in the mouth before the impression is taken, and the technique of bending the clasp is exactly as described previously. This may be either a single clasp or a double clasp, as shown in figure 69. In the double crib clasp a slight modification is used. Instead of bending the gold clasp wire around one tooth, it is bent in the shape of an S, starting at the lingual surface of one of the teeth to be clasped, continuing to the proximal surface of the tooth, and crossing the embrasure between

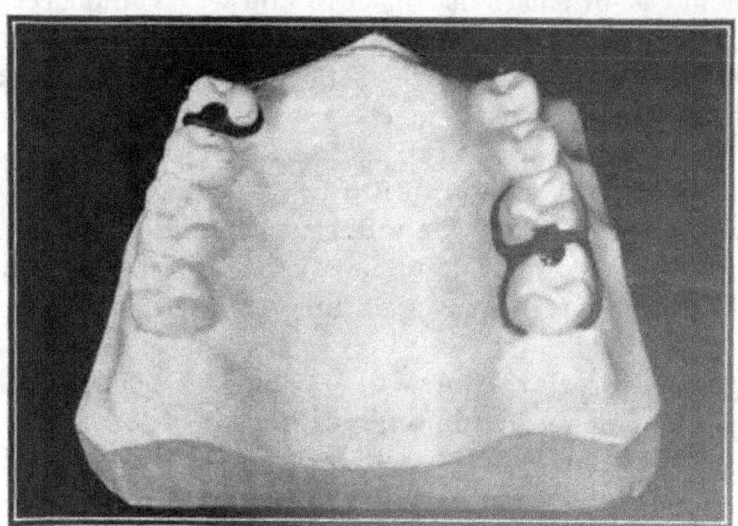

FIGURE 69.

the teeth, as described. But instead of continuing around the buccal of the same tooth, it is bent so as to form the buccal arm of the clasp for the other tooth to be clasped. When this S-shaped wire is formed, two other pieces of wire are bent to complete the unfinished arms of the clasp. These pieces are soldered to the S-shaped wire in their correct positions, thus completing the double crib clasp. Always construct an occlusal rest for all crib clasps in order to prevent the wire from separating the teeth, thus endangering their continued usefulness.

77. Cast clasps.—The designs as already given for wrought clasps will also apply to cast clasps. Frequently in the designing of partial dentures this is the type indicated. The impression of the teeth to be clasped is usually taken in plaster or hydrocolloid impression material. The impression is boxed in either moldine, if a metal model is to made, or wax, if the model is to be poured with investment plaster. The fit of the clasp is usually more accurate when cast directly on the investment plaster model. Therefore this will be the technique described herein. The outline of the clasp is traced on the model by the dental officer. A piece of 30-gage basewax is wrapped around the tooth and sealed with a warm spatula so that it will not move from position. The outline of the clasp which shows through the wax is then covered with a thin layer of either green or blue casting wax. After applying the wax, it is carved and smoothed to the shape of the clasp, which should also include the tail portion or that part that is to be used for anchorage. It is much easier to cast the tailpiece as part of the clasp than to make it of wire and then solder the two parts together. This anchorage should be of sufficient length to allow maximum retention in the denture material and should be made in the form of a loop to facilitate this retention. The outline of this loop should be marked on the model at the same time that the clasp is outlined and the waxing done as the clasp is waxed. When the wax clasp and tailpiece are carved and smoothed, the case is sprued by attaching a tapered wire such as a phonograph needle to the wax clasp, and holding it in place until it has cooled sufficiently to secure it. The clasp can then be invested and cast the same as any gold inlay or three-quarter crown. (See sec. IX.)

78. **Lingual and palatal bars.**—*a*. A lingual bar consists of a connecting piece of material running adjacent to the soft tissue on the linqual side of the lower front teeth beneath the tip of the tongue, joining the two sides of a lower partial denture and making it one unit. Palatal bars may be defined as metal bars constructed to fit the surface of the vault of the palate and connecting the two lateral sections of an upper partial denture. Lingual bars may be obtained in a ready-made form and all that is required is to adapt it to the individual model. However, in a few cases this is not entirely satisfactory, and it is better to cast the lingual bar as well as the palatal bar for these cases. The design of the bar is drawn on the model with an indelible pencil by the dental officer. It is frequently necessary to place a strip of adhesive tape on the model to provide relief before adapting the wax. The outline of the bar on the model is oiled, and over this outline is adapted a piece of 30-gage baseplate wax. Blue inlay wax is melted and placed over this outline, which shows through the first layer of basewax. It is then trimmed and carved to the exact shape of the completed lingual bar (fig. 70).

b. After smoothing the wax it is sprued, removed from the cast, washed with green soap and water, invested, and cast in saddle and bar gold.

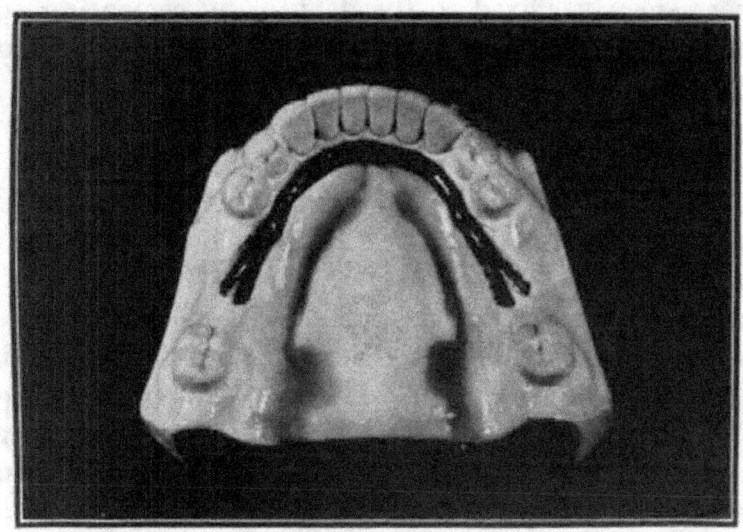

Figure 70.

Section XIV

CAST PARTIAL DENTURES AND PARTIAL DENTURE SKELETONS

	Paragraph
General	79
Models	80
Preparation of master model	81
Surveying model	82
Steps of survey	83
Location of retention	84
Eliminating undesirable undercuts	85
Tripoding	86
Duplicating model	87
Surveying casting model	88
Marking design on casting model	89
Waxing	90
Spruing	91
Investing	92
Burn-out and casting	93

79. General.—Many times it is desirable to cast the entire partial denture or a skeleton of the bars and clasps of the denture entirely in one piece. This type of partial denture makes a very fine restoration and the technique for its construction is very exacting. Where the entire partial denture is cast, a porcelain tooth, known as a tube tooth, is used. This tooth has a cylindrical cavity through the center which allows provision for its retention on the finished denture by means of a dowel or peg which is cast with the denture and on which the tube tooth fits. When the denture is finished, the tube teeth are permanently affixed to the denture by cementing them to place over the dowel with ordinary crown and bridge cement. In other cases, cast the bars and clasps of the denture joined with a skeletal framework. Vulcanite or other denture base material is later utilized to cover this framework and to attach the teeth to the partial denture. The two types of partial dentures are constructed in the same manner; that is, by casting them in one casting operation and in one piece.

80. **Models.**—A master model is obtained from the impression of the mouth. This master model is poured in stone as is described in paragraph 21. For this type of work a second model of casting investment must be obtained. This is accomplished by a process called duplicating the model. This second model is called a casting model as it is constructed of casting investment and is used directly in casting the partial denture.

81. **Preparation of master model.**—*a.* Designing the partial denture on the master model is the first step. The designing of the partial denture requires a direct knowledge of the condition found in the mouth of the patient. It also demands a knowledge of the effect of various forces on the various teeth and the tissue changes which are expected as a result of forces exerted. The dental mechanic is not required or expected to possess this knowledge, so the designing of the denture should be the work of the dental surgeon.

b. There are, however, a few fundamental facts which the dental mechanic should know. The two forces involved for which provision must be made in designing a denture, are—

(1) *Down pressure* against the ridges and remaining teeth brought to bear by the opposing jaw in closing the mouth. This pressure is sustained by occlusal rests on the denture which are little fingers fitting onto the occlusal surface of remaining natural teeth and are in most cases incorporated with each clasp. Paragraph 74 describes and illustrates one type of occlusal rest.

(2) *Up pressure* away from the ridges, which tends to unseat the denture. This is caused by sticky food, the weight of the appliance if in the upper jaw, etc. Up pressure is resisted by the retentive power of the clasps and by indirect retainers (finger projections which prevent tipping).

c. Three points firmly held on any object will in turn firmly hold that object. If three points (not in a straight line) are fixed firmly, the denture will be held securely. Usually then three clasps are needed to hold the denture in place. In order to prevent movement of the teeth, settling and displacement, the following must be observed: the denture must hold the abutment teeth rigidly in place, be rigid itself, and be solidly supported so that it will not rock or tilt. If the soft tissue, as well as the remaining teeth, is utilized in the support of the denture, wrought wire clasps or stress breakers should be employed to equalize the forces between the semirigid teeth and the semisoft tissue. This problem will not be discussed in this manual as it is the prerogative of the dental surgeon and out of the field of the technician.

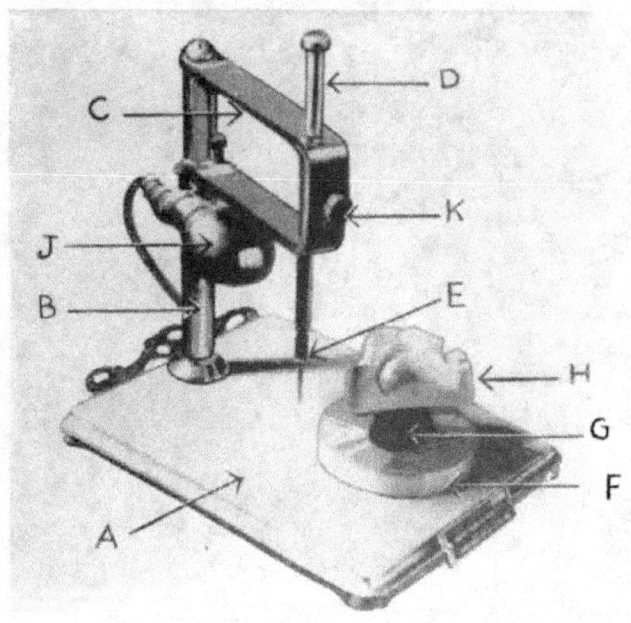

A. Flat base.
B. Vertical member.
C. Horizontal arm.
E. Carbon point for marking model.
F. Movable base for mounting cast.
G. Mounting wax.
H. Cast.
K. Lock nut.

FIGURE 71.—Surveying instrument.

82. Surveying model.—Before the design is drawn in pencil on the model, the exact design of the clasps is determined. This is done with the aid of a surveying instrument (fig. 71) which marks the height of contour of each tooth surface. With the relative points of highest contour marked as a line on each tooth to be clasped, the outline of the clasp may be accurately drawn on the tooth. In this type of work it is necessary to obtain such accuracy in the design of each clasp. The reason is that these cast clasps are more rigid than the wire clasps taken up in section XIII and their success depends upon their accuracy in design.

83. Steps of survey.—The surveying instrument (fig. 71) consists of a flat base A, a metallic disk which is placed on the base F, an upright supporting a horizontal arm C, which in turn supports the vertical member containing a carbon point E for marking the model.

a. The model is mounted on the metallic disk by means of a ball of wax as shown in figure 72. It is placed on the wax in the position which will afford desirable undercuts on the abutment teeth for the clasps. This may be determined by looking down on the model from above while adjusting it.

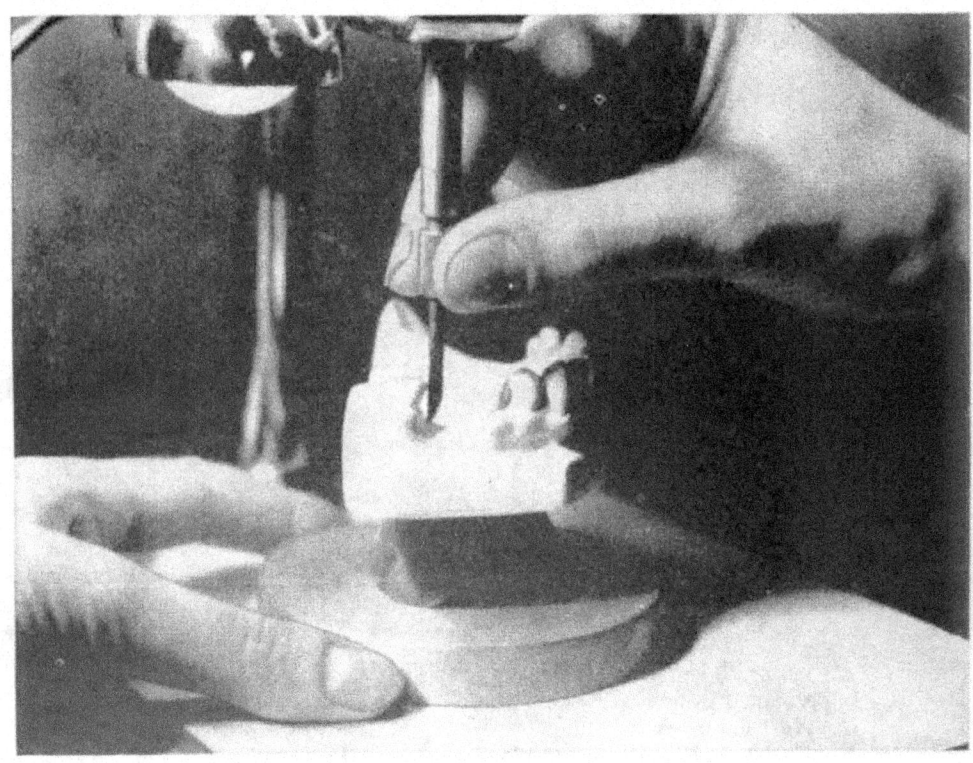

FIGURE 72.—Marking line of greatest circumference on tooth to be clasped.

b. The vertical side of the carbon is placed against each tooth that may be involved in the case, and it is moved around all surfaces of these teeth by moving the movable base F and by swinging the horizontal arm C to facilitate this. The circumference of greatest contour is located wherever the vertical side of the surveying tool touches the tooth. Wherever light shows between the tool and the tooth below this circumference the undercut area is located. The carbon point will effectively mark this line of greatest circumference on the tooth.

84. Location of retention.—By this procedure the desirable and ndesirable undercuts immediately show up. The teeth to be used for retention can quickly be determined. If possible these teeth should be well-formed, strong, and widely distributed in the mouth.

85. **Eliminating undesirable undercuts.**—The undercuts which show up after surveying will be used largely in designing the clasps so that they provide retention for those clasps. However, in some places, especially on the surfaces of the teeth adjoining the edentulous spaces, undercuts are not desired. Construction of the denture into these undercut areas would prevent its going to place. These undercuts are eliminated by filling them with wax on the master model (fig. 73). In this way, in the next step (duplicating the model) these undesirable undercuts will not appear on the casting model.

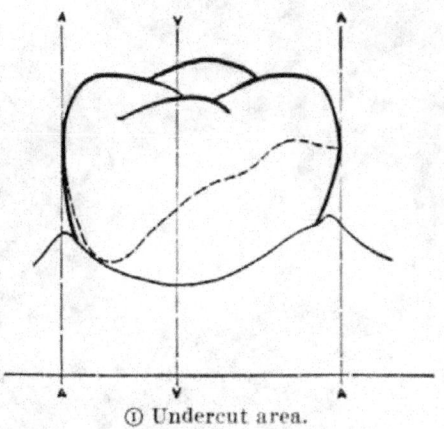

① Undercut area.

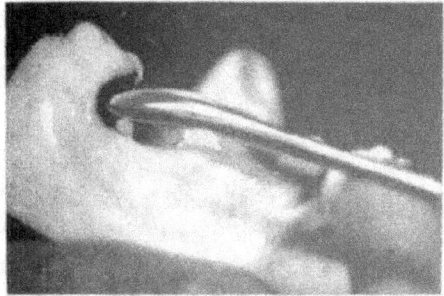

② Placing wax in undercut.

FIGURE 73.—Filling in undesirable undercut with wax.

86. **Tripoding.**—Before removing the master model from the mounting wax, a determination of its position must be made so that the investment model may be placed back on the surveyor in the same position as the master model. This procedure is called tripoding. In order to tripod, it is only necessary to determine three points in the same horizontal plane on the master model. This is done by locking the spindle in position by using the lock nut (fig. 71, *K*),

placing a drop of ink on the tip of the surveying tool, and touching the model at three points. These three points will be in a plane parallel to the fixed base.

87. Duplicating model.—After surveying the master model, drawing the design on the master model in pencil, and filling the undesirable undercuts on the model with wax, a casting model can then be made. This step is called duplicating the model.

a. Soak the master model in water for a short period of time.

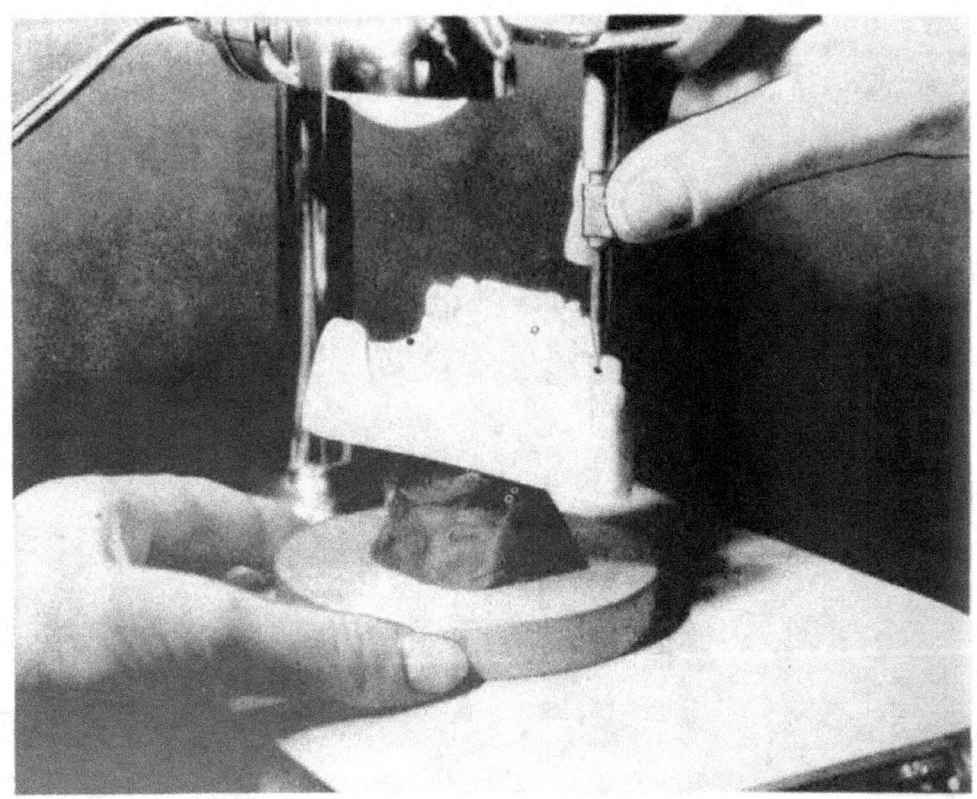

FIGURE 74.—Marking three points with tip of tool so that duplicate model can be replaced on conveyor in same plane.

b. Touch the three tripod points with an indelible pencil after soaking the model.

c. Place the master model in a duplicating flask. Several flasks are on the market for this purpose. However, if none are obtainable a small can with top and bottom removed can be used by placing over the model after the model has been fixed to a flat surface.

d. Hydrocolloid impression material is prepared by heating in a hydrocolloid heater or an ordinary double boiler. Old impressions and scrap pieces are best for this if an equal volume of water is added before heating. As soon as the material begins to boil, stir to facilitate an even mix.

e. Let the hydrocolloid material cool to the proper consistency before pouring (140° F.). Pour the material first around the sides of the model and then all over it, completely filling the flask or can. After the hydrocolloid material has completely set (15 to 30 minutes) invert the flask or can and gently remove the master model.

f. Dry out the excess water from the impression and *immediately* pour an investment model of any model investment. This same material will later be used to invest the case for actual casting.

g. Before pouring the investment, it should be noted that the tripod marks appear on the impression. These should be touched with indelible pencil so that they will carry through into the investment model. The model investment should be thoroughly mixed to obtain its maximum strength. The use of measuring cups and mechanical mixer is highly recommended. As soon as the investment is poured, dust some dry investment powder on the back of the model to draw out the excess water.

h. Allow the investment to set for 1 hour in the hydrocolloid. The hydrocolloid should then be broken away from the investment. Do not attempt to save the impression by pulling the investment model out in the same manner that the master model was removed, as the freshly set surface of the investment may be marred by the friction. It will be found that the tripod marks now appear on the investment model.

88. Surveying casting model.—After the casting model is thoroughly dry, mount it on the mounting wax, manipulate the model until the three tripod points can be touched by the tip of the surveying tool without raising or lowering the spindle. In other words, arrange the model so that the three tripod points will be a plane parallel with the fixed base. The investment model will now be in exactly the same tilted position as the master model was when surveyed. Mark the circumference on the teeth to be clasped on the casting model and remove from instrument.

89. Marking design on casting model.—The denture design decided upon on the master model is now traced out in pencil on the casting model. The exact outline of the clasps, with the aid of the survey marks, are placed on the model. This outline of the design should be done by the dental officer.

90. Waxing.—Generally, ordinary blue casting wax is used. It is applied to the model in a molten state with a spatula and later trimmed to the desired shape and size with wax-carving instruments. Thin sheet wax, where available, may be used in places where saddles are being constructed. In this way the desired thickness is more accurately determined than if the inlay wax were applied. Also, wax shapes are supplied in proper sizes for clasps and bars; these may be used if available. The waxing step is important and should be carefully done so that little grinding will be necessary after the denture is cast.

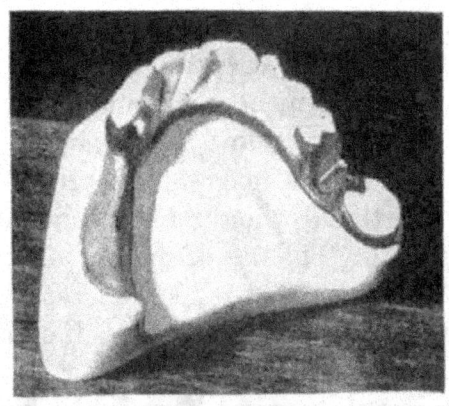

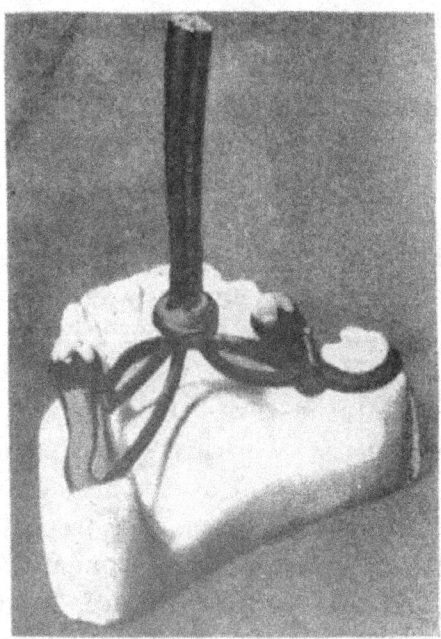

FIGURE 75.—Wax pattern on model and wax pattern sprued ready for investment.

91. Spruing.—Sprues are distributed about the case. Usually one sprue to the body of the partial below each clasp will be sufficient. In long saddle areas it is well to place one sprue at each end of the saddle. It is not advisable to attach a sprue to a bar or clasp as the point where the sprue attaches is usually a weak spot in the denture. Three sprues in most cases are enough. The sprues are joined about ¼ inch above the highest point of the pattern and sealed together. Above this point the sprues are sealed together to provide one large sprue (fig. 75).

92. Investing.—Such large castings are best invested by first coating all parts of the pattern with investment and bringing well up on the sprue. A second batch is then mixed to insert the previously coated pattern in the investment ring. First the invested model with the sprued pattern is soaked well in a pan of water. Next, a generous coat of investment is painted on the pattern, and finally a second batch of investment is mixed and the coated model is placed in the ring. A crucible is cut in the investment after the investing material sets.

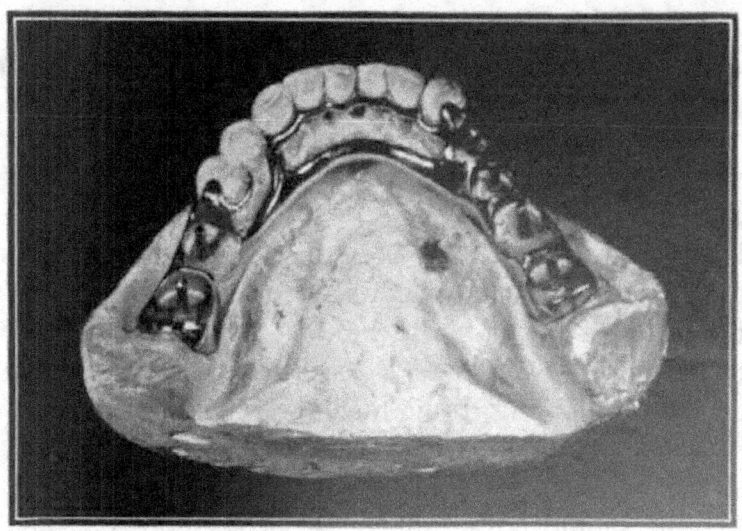

FIGURE 76.—Finished cast ready for cementation of porcelain tube teeth.

93. Burn-out and casting.—After the investment has set 45 minutes, it is placed in the furnace to burn out the wax. The casting is made as described in section IX. The gold should be melted in the casting machine while the flask is still in the furnace. This will prevent the cooling of the case while melting the large amount of gold necessary for casting. Allow the investment to stand 4 or 5 minutes after casting and then plunge in water. When cold, dig and brush the investment away from the casting. The casting is pickled and finished in the usual way. The master model is utilized in fitting, finishing, and polishing the casting. Figure 76 shows a finished cast gold partial denture on the master model; tube teeth fit over the dowels and later will be cemented.

Section XV

SPLINTS

	Paragraph
General	94
Vulcanite splint	95
Acrylic resin splint	96
Cast silver splint	97

94. General.—Splints are becoming more and more important in the Army dental service. In warfare, injuries to the face and jaws are very common, and are becoming increasingly so. The most practical method of controlling fractures of the jaw is by splinting. It must be understood that no two cases will be the same or will use exactly the same design of splint, but they are all sufficiently similar to follow the same general basic fundamentals of design and construction. The following designs can be used for either maxillary or mandibular splints and can be constructed of vulcanite, acrylic resin, or cast silver. The variations in material and design will be taken up in detail.

95. Vulcanite splint (fig. 77).—*a.* The prepared model will come to the dental technician for the construction of the splint.

b. The designing of the case will be done by the dental officer and will be outlined on the model. It is important that the dental technician know the following fundamentals in the designing of all splints so that the maximum efficiency and serviceability will be obtained.

(1) The splint should cover all free gingival margins on the lingual, buccal, and labial surfaces at least 2 or 3 millimeters from the necks of the teeth.

(2) The splint must cover the cervical two-thirds of the teeth and must include as much of the occlusal third as possible without interfering with the masticatory processes.

c. Adapt a piece of 28-gage casting wax to the model to cover the design of the splint. Make certain the wax is in all the interproximal spaces.

d. Soften a piece of baseplate wax and fold it over on itself, making a double thickness. Adapt this wax over the wax already in place, on both the lingual and buccal surfaces of the cast. Trim wax to conform with design of splint, as outlined on the cast.

e. Make a small button of the labial surface of the wax pattern in the median line. This wax button may be stamped out of a piece of wax, using a lead pencil from which the rubber has been removed.

DENTAL TECHNICIANS

This small disk is attached to the wax pattern, forming the small button which will be used to secure the finished splint in place in the mouth.

f. The edges of the wax must be sealed to the model.

g. Chill the wax in cold water and polish with cotton.

h. Flame the wax and repolish, which will give a very smooth finish to the splint and will minimize the amount of polishing to be done later.

i. A piece of 14-gage half-round wire is bent to conform to the distal surface of the last molar tooth. It extends forward on both the lingual and buccal surfaces of the tooth, only touching the tooth on the distal surface. The ends should come forward to almost the mesial of the tooth and then bend out at right angles, extending beyond the surface of the wax pattern. These two projections of the wire, along with that portion around the distal of the tooth, will be imbedded in plaster during the flasking process, thus holding the wire in its correct position.

j. In some fractures, it is necessary to design the case so that a loose or broken fragment of bone in an area which is edentulous may be held in place. This is accomplished by constructing projections of wire which will extend out from the splint and hold these fragments in place. A piece of nickel tubing 10- by 14-gage is incorporated into the splint by soldering it to the buccal surface of the half-round wire, so that it will be parallel to the buccal surface of the teeth. A piece of 14-gage square wire is inserted into the tubing and the other end is bent so that it will rest on the buccal tissue over the fragment requiring stabilization.

k. Wax is melted around the nickel tubing so that it is flush with the surface of the wax pattern.

l. The case is now ready for flasking. Trim off all occlusal surfaces of the teeth flush with the wax pattern. Soak the model in cold water until all bubbling has ceased. Flask the case in the lower part of the flask, as described in section VI, making certain that the plaster comes up to the lower border of the wax splint. The tubing and wires are left exposed. Use any type of separating medium on the plaster surface and then pour the upper half of the flask, as previously described.

m. The wax is eliminated, the case is packed with rubber, vulcanized, and polished, as previously described.

n. In every space where there is a tooth missing the buccal and lingual parts of the splint are separated by sawing. The button in the median line is also sawed vertically in half. Thus, the splint is in two parts connected by wire, which can be placed in the mouth, brought into position, and the two halves of the button wired together.

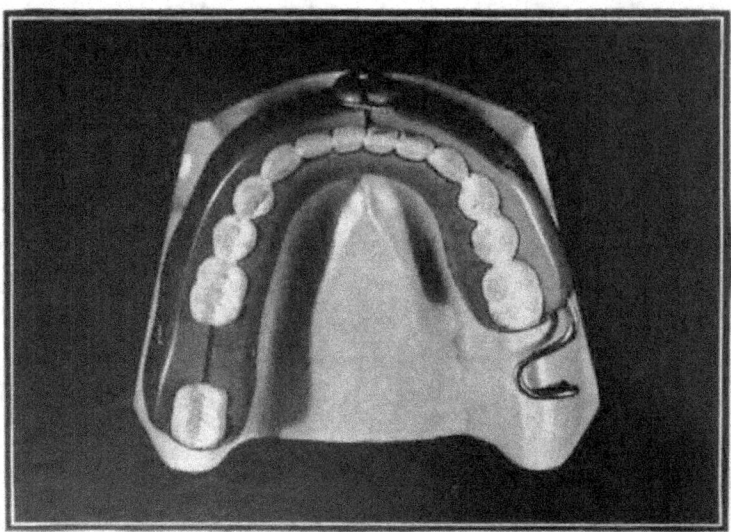

FIGURE 77.—Vulcanite splint with posterior extension arm for stabilizing posterior fragment.

96. **Acrylic resin splint.**—The construction of a splint, using the acrylic resin material in place of the vulcanite, is exactly the same as previously described with the exception of tinfoiling the wax pattern and the model. This tinfoiling procedure is carried

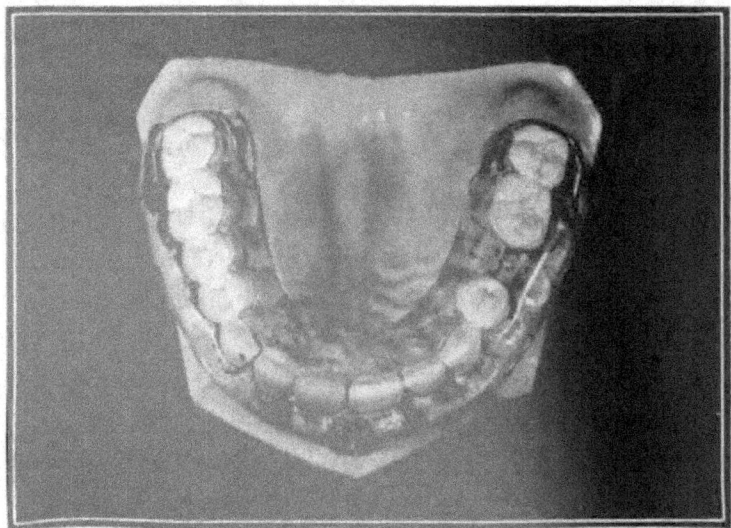

FIGURE 78.—Acrylic resin splint.

out the same as already described under acrylic resin dentures. The acrylic resin used in the construction of the splints is colorless, which has the advantage of being transparent, allowing the dental officer to observe the condition of the teeth and gums underlying the splint at all times. Frequently a fracture case will have one or two missing anterior teeth. It is a simple procedure to add the necessary artificial teeth to the splint, which will replace the missing teeth until the splint can be removed. When teeth are added, it is necessary to tinfoil over the labial surfaces of the artificial teeth before the case is waxed. This will prevent the material from adhering to the labial surfaces of the teeth. Acrylic resin splint showing teeth added is illustrated in figure 78.

97. Cast silver splint.—*a.* The third type of splint that is commonly used is the cast silver splint.

(1) Prepare a duplicate model of investment plaster.

(2) Adapt one thickness of 28-gage wax to the investment plaster model as outlined by the dental officer.

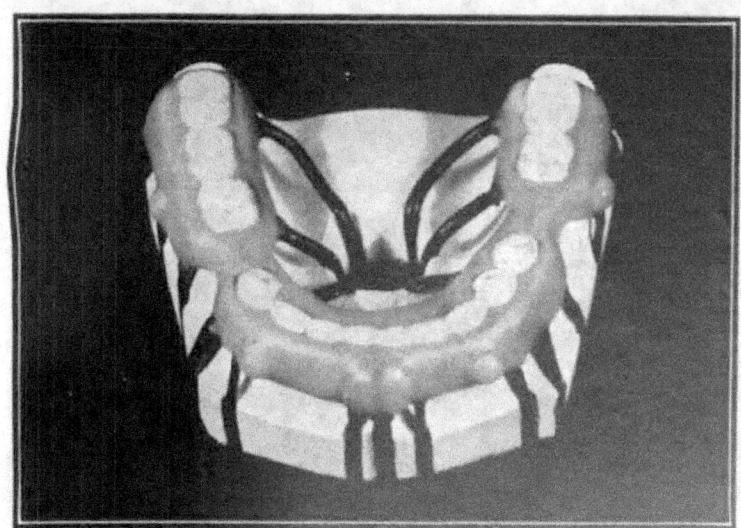

FIGURE 79.—Wax pattern on model and sprued for casting splint in silver.

(3) Soften a piece of baseplate wax and adapt *one* thickness of it over the wax already in place.

(4) Add sufficient wax so that the surface of the wax pattern is smooth and even.

(5) Fourteen-gage wire is used, as previously described.

(6) The button in the median line is constructed as usual and smaller buttons are placed in the cuspid and first molar region of both sides.

(7) Seal the edges of the wax to the model.

(8) Smooth and polish the pattern as this will save needless work in the final polishing.

(9) There are various ways of spruing the case preparatory to investing and casting, but the method described in this manual will

be found very satisfactory. Drill a hole through the center of the model about the size of a dime. On the inner lingual surface of the pattern are attached six small 14-gage sprues. On the outer surface leading from the main sprue are attached four 14-gage sprues attached to the buccal surface of the wax pattern. From the cuspid

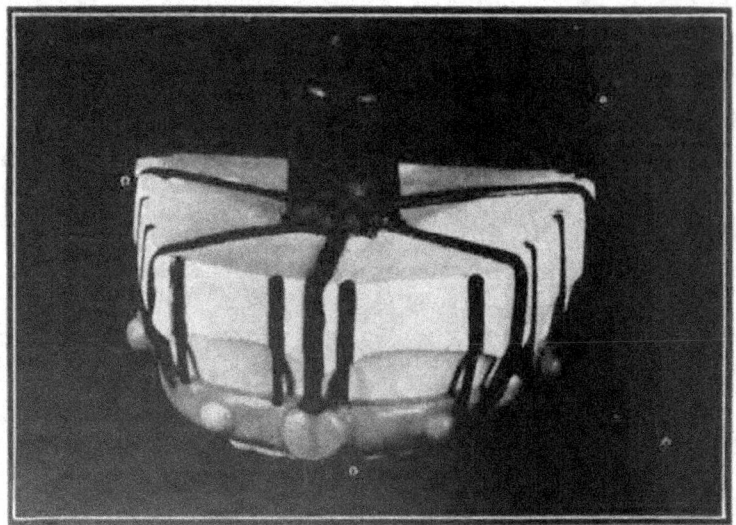

FIGURE 80.—Another view of wax pattern for silver splint.

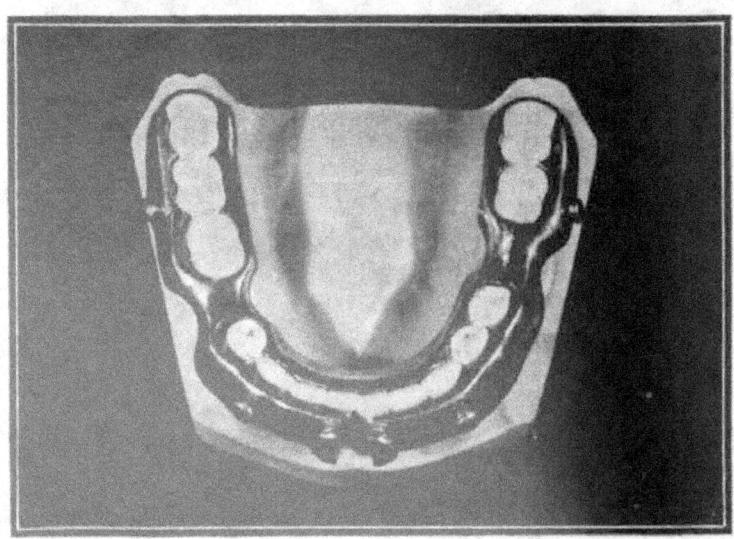

FIGURE 81.—Finished silver splint.

and molar regions of the buccal surface of the pattern are attached 14-gage sprues for air vents. These air vents stop at the edge of the model. Grooves should be cut in the model, both lingual and buccal, to accommodate these sprues (figs. 79 and 80).

    b. Soak model until bubbling ceases. Using a camel's-hair brush, paint wax pattern with casting investment, making certain that all air bubbles are eliminated. Select casting ring to fit the case and fill with remaining investment. Place the model in the investment with the teeth down and the main sprue which comes through the hole in the center of the model sticking out of the investment material. Let set for at least 1 hour. Place casting ring in cold oven and heat for 2 hours at 1,200° F. Add not more than 10 percent copper to the amount of silver. Melt silver and copper in crucible. Place ring in casting machine. Add borax or any reducing flux to molten metal and cast. Remove from investment and polish. Make cuts the same as previously described. A finished splint is shown in figure 81.

Chapter 4

DENTAL X-RAY TECHNICIAN

		Paragraphs
Section	I. Equipment	98–103
	II. Intra-oral roentgenography	104–125
	III. Extra-oral roentgenography	126–129
	IV. Processing of X-ray films	130–138

Section I

EQUIPMENT

	Paragraph
General	98
Dental X-ray machine	99
Films	100
Emulsion	101
Physics	102
Intensifying screen	103

98. General.—The Army dental surgeon, in connection with routine professional procedures, is called upon to make numerous and varied dental surveys; surveys for evidence of dental foci of infection; surveys in connection with different boards requiring physical examinations of the individuals; annual and semiannual surveys; surveys of commands, etc. Each of these is of particular value in connection with the regulation requiring the examination. Therefore, the findings must be accurately recorded and reported as indicated. The survey for evidence of dental foci of infection is of particular importance in connection with general and localized conditions that may be attributed to or influenced by oral or dental foci. Good roentgenographic studies are of inestimable value in connection with a thorough clinical examination in order that a complete and correct oral diagnostic report can be rendered. Roentgenographic studies include roentgenograms, or X-rays as commonly called, plain and stereoscopic views, also fluoroscopic observations. The images or shadows shown on the film and those viewed on the fluoroscopic screen should be clearly and sharply outlined, giving good detail and contrast. The correct interpretation of these studies, in connection with the clinical examination, will greatly assist the operator in locating and viewing the normal as well as abnormal conditions. The opportunity to see the parts in X-ray studies is of material aid in rendering a diagnosis of invisible conditions. Therefore, it is evident that the real value of X-ray studies as diagnostic aids will be in direct proportion to their quality.

99. Dental X-ray machine.—The majority of dental X-ray machines are shockproof and, with few exceptions, have oil immersed tubes. The head is small and mounted so that adjustment of position is easily accomplished. The newer machines are capable of adjustment of voltage, kilovoltage, and milliamperage. The panel is located on the top of the cabinet and for adjustment has "on" and "off" switch, control knob to adjust the voltage so that the specified voltage for that machine is registered on the voltmeter when the machine is in operation, knobs to adjust the kilovoltage from 50 to 70 kilovolts, and another knob to control milliamperes which are recorded on a milliammeter.

100. Films.—Films for roentgenographic work are supplied in various sizes and usually a dozen or more are in each container. Storage is important, and a lead-lined box or chest should be provided in which unexposed and undeveloped films can be kept to protect them from radiation. The storage should be in a cool, dry place; high temperatures, moisture, chemicals, or the like deteriorate or ruin the emulsion of the films for X-ray work. An expiration date is stamped on each package indicating the manufacturer's time limit on the emulsion. Films should not be overstocked. Sufficient films should always be on hand, but in such quantities that they will be used within the expiration date. However, films stored and protected as outlined should produce satisfactory X-rays long after the expiration date.

101. Emulsion.—*a.* The emulsion referred to is the dull surface side of the film, and in case of a duplitized film both sides are coated. This emulsion is a thin coating of special gelatin in which the minute particles of sensitive silver halide salts are incorporated. The base on which the emulsion is placed is a transparent cellulose acetate support with a slight bluish tint or color. Films that do not have this bluish tint or color may be viewed over tinted ground glass, giving better photographic effect.

b. Films for X-ray, like those for photography, have various emulsion speeds indicating their sensitivity to radiation. The terms used for marking the speed of X-ray films are regular, medium, fast, extrafast, or similar words indicating the emulsion's sensitivity to radiation. The effect of developing solutions on the emulsion is discussed in section IV. Extra-fast dental films require about 75 percent less exposure time than regular films to give the same photographic effect, other factors being equal. The duplitized will require 50 percent less time than the regular to obtain the same results. An example would be 2 seconds for extra-fast, 4 seconds for duplitized, and 8 seconds for regular. The more important factors that influence and affect the production of the image or shadow (photographic effect) on the emulsion are: kilovoltage, milliamperage, target film distance, object film distance, thickness and density of the object, emulsion speed of the film, intensifying screen speed, and processing. It is evident that a good roentgenogram will be the result of an exacting technique and from this there must be no deviation. Sufficient exposures should be made and the factors governing photographic effect considered until the X-rays produced are up to a high standard. An exposure chart can then be made that will give the technician information on that equipment and assure him of producing films of satisfactory quality.

102. Physics.—It is not the purpose of this manual to go into too much detail as to the physics of the X-ray machine, but rather the technique involved in its handling so that the technician will be able to take consistently good pictures. The X-ray technician may be called upon to understand and operate several types of units. They may vary, but it is believed the technique described in this manual will give the technician sufficient knowledge to operate the various makes of dental X-ray apparatus and obtain excellent results.

a. Voltage.—When the switch is turned to "on," the voltage is registered on the voltmeter. The line voltage should register 110 volts on the voltmeter when the machine is in operation. Some machines advise adjustment of the voltage for exposures made at 10 milliamperes and 15 milliamperes, with a line on the voltmeter indicating each. The manufacturer's instructions for each machine should be followed.

b. Kilovoltage.—Machines with variable kilovoltage have adjustments from 50 to 70 kilovolts. This factor is the driving or rather penetrating power of the rays. The use of higher kilovoltage gives more penetration of the bones or tissues being exposed, resulting in more rays reaching the film which gives it a flat appearance lacking in contrast. Therefore, lower kilovoltage will produce a film with greater contrast.

c. Milliamperage.—The milliamperes can be regulated by adjusting the resistance unit of that circuit. Dental machines usually operate on 10 or 15 milliamperes and as a rule should not be used below 6 or above 15. The time of exposure in seconds multiplied by the number of milliamperes, as shown by the milliammeter, gives the number of milliampere seconds. For example, 4 seconds of exposure using 10 milliamperes equals 40 milliampere seconds. The dose necessary to produce erythema causing a temporary redness of the skin is approximately 1,200 milliampere seconds at a target distance of 8 inches. At 16 inches, it would be 4,800 milliampere seconds. It has been suggested that operators never exceed one-half the erythema dose, or 600 milliampere seconds. If this limit is exceeded, it may subject the patient to grave danger. If the patient states that he has been subjected recently to considerable radiation, the examination should be deferred until 3 weeks after the last exposure. Two complete dental surveys of 16 exposures each may be safely made as it will be well within the safety limit. However, if skull pictures, sinuses, or facial bones are to be exposed in addition to the dental survey, consideration should be given to avoid overexposure of the patient in a 3-week period.

d. Target film distance.—A uniform target film distance is essential to produce films of uniform density. To effect this, always place the cone of the machine in close proximity to the patient's face when making intra-oral exposures. This automatically adjusts the target distance at 8 inches, the distance recommended for most dental machines. If greater target film distance is desired the tip of the cone may be placed 1, 2, or 3 inches from the skin surface.

e. Rays.—The tip of the cone acts as the guide in determining the direction of the rays or beams of radiation, as it is always in alinement with the target of the tube. The correct angle of the rays is most important as this will distribute the flow of radiation evenly over the area to be exposed.

f. Precautions.—Under no circumstances should the operator hold the films in the patient's mouth. This is to be done by the patient. In those cases where it is impossible for the patient to hold the films, the film packet may be grasped with a hemostat and held by an assistant from such a position that he will not be in the line of exposure. During the exposure, the operator should place himself as far away from the unit as possible. If a large number of roentgenograms are to be taken daily, he should protect himself by placing a lead screen between himself and the unit. It must be remembered that carelessness on the part of the operator in this matter will cause overexposure of himself or his assistant and possibly with serious results. If precautions are taken, the operator has nothing to fear, although the machine may be in frequent use.

103. **Intensifying screen.**—Due to the fact that less than 1 percent of the X-ray energy is absorbed by the sensitized film emulsion in the formation of the image, a device known as the intensifying screen has been developed to utilize the wasted rays so that the exposure time may be reduced. The screen consists of a flexible but substantial cardboard coated with finely divided crystals of calcium tungstate. Two of these screens are mounted in a cassette designed to hold the film between them during the exposure. The loading of

the cassette must be done in a dark room. *The black piece of paper must be removed* from around the film when using the intensifying screen; otherwise, the result is about the same as though the screens were not used.

Section II

INTRA-ORAL ROENTGENOGRAPHY

	Paragraph
Vertical angle	104
Horizontal angle	105
Position of head	106
Interproximal or bite-wing examination	107
Molar and bicuspid	108
Central, lateral, and canine	109
Periapical examination	110
Maxillary molar	111
Maxillary bicuspid	112
Maxillary canine	113
Maxillary incisor	114
Mandibular molar	115
Mandibular bicuspid	116
Mandibular canine	117
Mandibular incisor	118
Occlusal examination	119
Maxillary occlusal (full view)	120
Maxillary central and lateral incisor	121
Maxillary canine, bicuspid, and molar	122
Mandibular central and lateral incisor	123
Mandibular canine, bicuspid, and molar	124
Mandibular occlusal (full view)	125

104. Vertical angle.—In making dental roentgenograms, it is usually necessary to direct the rays upon structures that lie at an angle with the film. If the following rule is strictly adhered to, approximately correct images of the teeth can be recorded on the film: direct the rays from the tube so that they will be perpendicular to the plane that bisects the angle formed by the long axis of the tooth and the plane of the film packet (fig. 82). Any deviation from this will result in the image either being elongated or shortened.

a. In figure 83 the rays are striking the film from too low an angle with the result that the image of the tooth is lengthened as shown.

b. In figure 84 the rays are striking the film from too high an angle with the result that the image of the tooth is shortened.

c. In figure 85 the rays are striking the film from the correct angle; that is, they are striking the film perpendicularly to the bisecting plane midway between the film and the tooth. This results

DENTAL TECHNICIANS TM 8-225
104

in the image of the tooth being imposed upon the film in the correct proportion.

d. This applies mostly to the maxillary teeth due to the palatal arch, although it also applies to the lower anterior teeth. The lower molar teeth do not present this problem as the film can usually

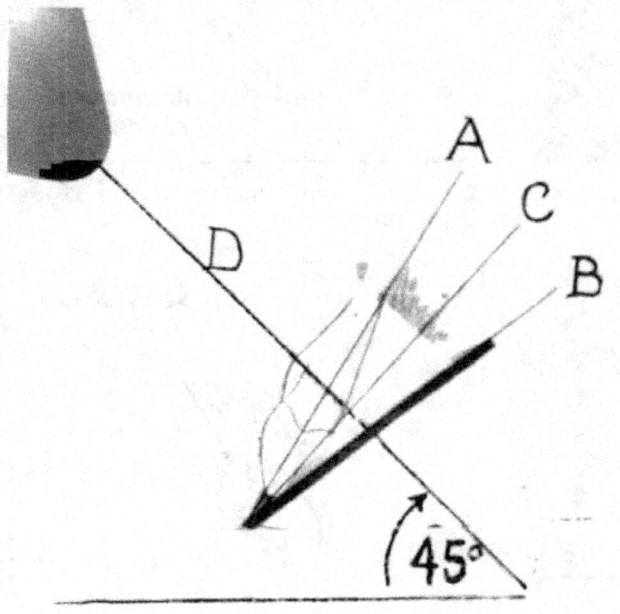

FIGURE 82.—Correct projection angle for maxillary canine.

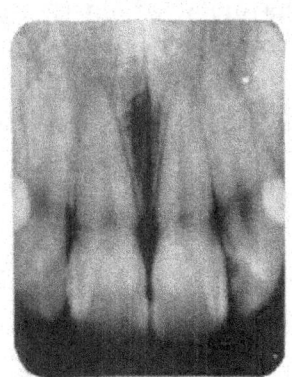
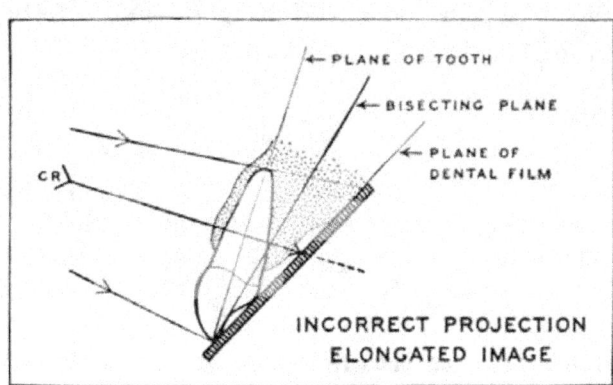

FIGURE 83.—Roentgen rays striking film from too low an angle. Tooth image lengthened in resulting roentgenogram.

be placed in such a position that it is nearly parallel to the long axis of the teeth. Thus the rays can be directed almost perpendicularly to both the teeth and the film.

e. The vertical angles will vary in different cases and certain modifications of angles must be made accordingly. The following

107

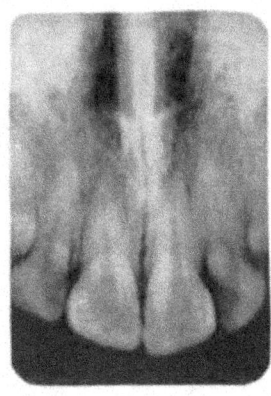 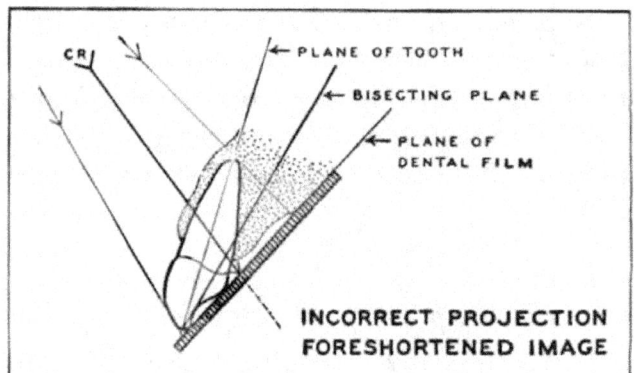

FIGURE 84.—Roentgen rays striking film from too high an angle. Tooth image shortened in resulting roentgenogram.

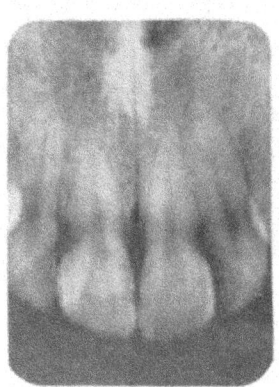 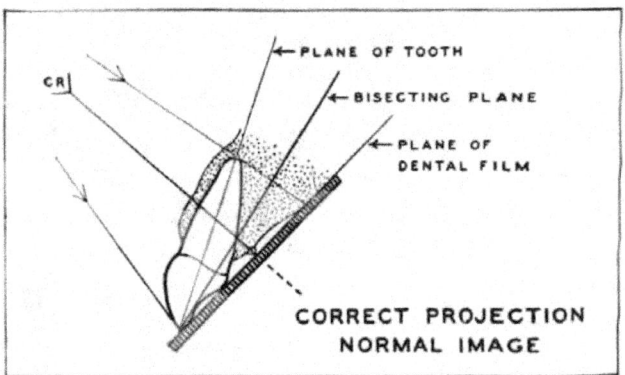

FIGURE 85.—Roentgen rays striking film from correct angle. Tooth image in correct proportions.

table, however, is a usable guide and in the majority of cases will give good results:

Upper	Degrees	Lower	Degrees
Molars	+20	Molars	−5
Bicuspids	+30	Bicuspids	−10
Canine	+45	Canine	−20
Centrals	+40	Centrals	−15

105. **Horizontal angle.**—*a.* If the horizontal angle is not correct the result will be an overlapping of the images of the crowns of the teeth. When this occurs, the chief value of the X-ray is gone as two of the most important areas to be examined are distorted, namely, the contact point between the teeth and the periodontal membrane surrounding the roots of the teeth. This error is illustrated in figure 86.

b. To obtain the correct direction of the rays in the horizontal plane, it must be directed through the teeth, parallel to the proximal surfaces and perpendicular to the antero-posterior plane of the film. This is illustrated in figure 86.

106. Position of head.—In this method where fixed angles are used, it is important to have the patient's head in a fixed position with

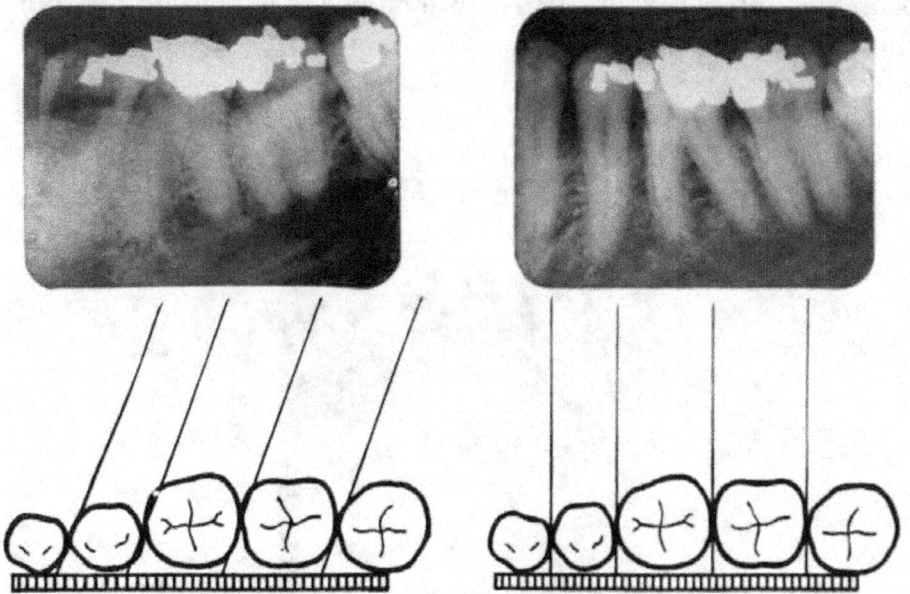

① Overlapping image caused by incorrect horizontal projection of rays. ② Correct image obtained by proper horizontal projection of rays.

FIGURE 86.

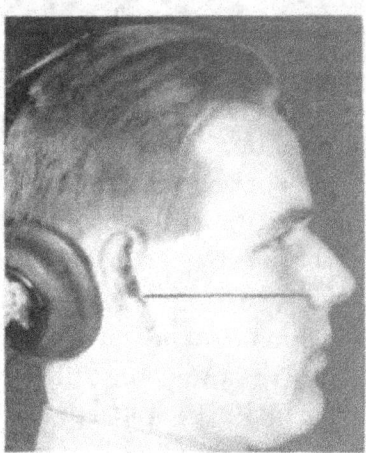

FIGURE 87.—Position of head with occlusal plane of upper arch horizontal.

the occlusal surfaces of the teeth to be X-rayed in a horizontal plane. Thus when the upper teeth are to be exposed, the occlusal surfaces of all the upper teeth should be horizontal. An imaginary line drawn from the tragus of the ear of the ala of the nose will act as a convenient guide line. This is illustrated in figure 87. The position of the head for exposing the lower teeth and having the occlusal surfaces horizontal is illustrated in figure 88. In this instance the imaginary line is drawn from the tragus of the ear to the angle of the mouth.

107. Interproximal or bite-wing examination.—The purpose of using the bite-wing film is to obtain an image of the coronal portion of the teeth without the distortion that usually occurs in a periapical examination. This is due to the fact that a low vertical angle of projection is used and the film packet is placed in a vertical position, permitting the X-rays to pass straight through the crowns of the teeth. This reveals areas that are obscured in the periapical roentgenograms where a high angle of projection on standard dental films is necessary.

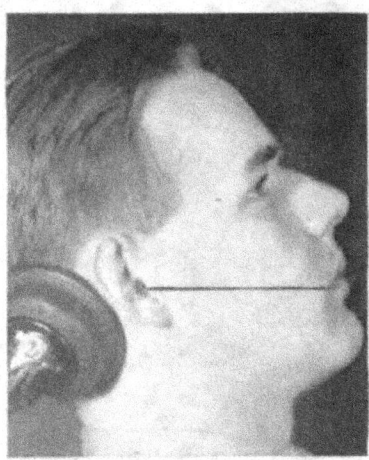

FIGURE 88.—Position of head with occlusal plane of lower arch horizontal.

108. Molar and bicuspid.—After adjusting the head so that the occlusal surfaces of the maxillary teeth are horizontal, place the bite-wing film packet in the patient's mouth so that the teeth when brought together will close on the wing, thus holding the film snugly against the lingual surfaces of the teeth. In a full mouth survey, it is best to start with the posterior teeth on one side and work around to the other side. Place the packet so that it will include the last tooth, guiding the lower part in first and then allow the upper part to slant into the palatal vault. Have the patient close normally. Incline the tube of the machine to a $+8°$ above horizontal and direct slightly disto-lingually so that the rays will pass straight through the interproximal spaces perpendicular to the plane of the film (fig. 89). For exposure time see chart at end of section.

109. Central, lateral, and canine.—Use an anterior bite-wing film for the examination of the incisor teeth. This differs from the posterior film in having its long axis in a vertical direction instead of a horizontal. Place the packet in the patient's mouth with the middle of the film on the median line. The lower part is guided into place, letting the upper part slant into the palatal vault. Have patient close, bringing the teeth end to end. For an examination of

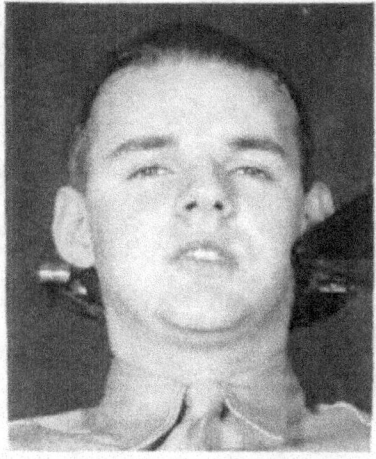
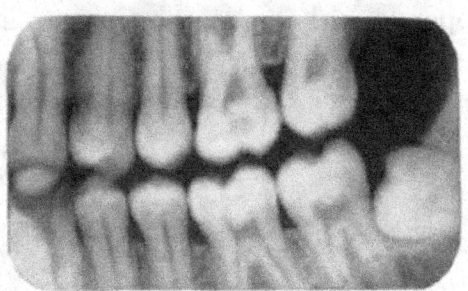

① Head position with occlusal plane of upper arch horizontal and tube inclined 8° above horizontal.

② Resulting bite-wing roentgenogram.

FIGURE 89.—Molar and bicuspid area.

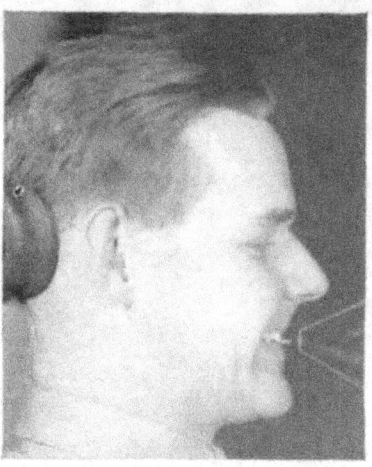

① Head position with occlusal plane of upper arch horizontal and tube inclined 8° above horizontal.

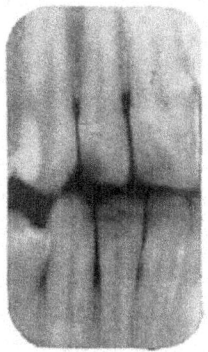 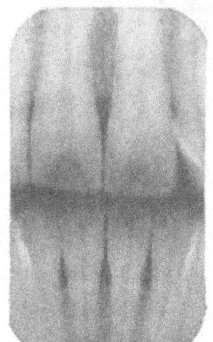 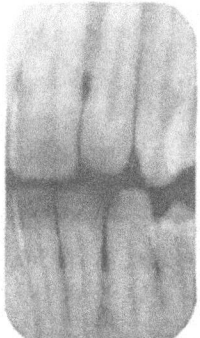

② Resulting bite-wing roentgenogram.

FIGURE 90.—Central, lateral, and canine areas.

the lateral-canine region, place the packet in the central region as described above, having the patient bite gently, then shift the wing distally until the mesial edge is even with the mesial surface of the central incisor. Have patient close teeth, end to end. Incline the tube 8° above horizontal, directing the rays straight through the upper lateral for lateral-canine region (fig. 90).

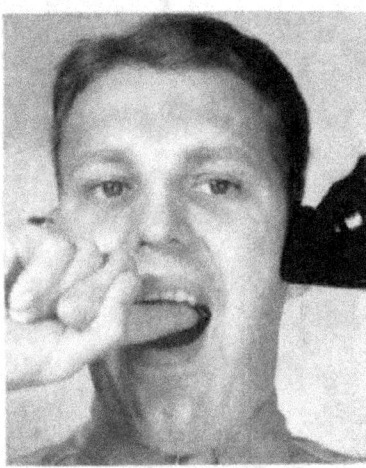

① Correct position of head, index finger, film, and tube.

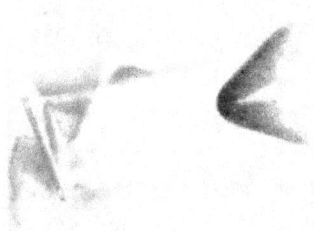

② Diagram of relation of rays to film. Tube inclined 20° above horizontal for average case.

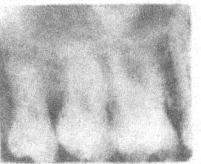

③ Resulting roentgenogram.
FIGURE 91.—Maxillary molar area.

110. **Periapical examination.**—These exposures are made on standard dental films with an increase in the vertical projection angle as compared with the bite-wing exposures. The images recorded are approximately their correct size, giving views of the periapical region, the teeth, and their supporting structures. A very complete dental survey can be made by using 14 standard dental films. Seven films

are used for each arch; two molar, two biscuspid, two canine, and one for the central area. Assuming that a full mouth roentgenographic examination is to be made, it is best to follow a definite sequence in taking the pictures so that the movements of the machine and the patient will be at a minimum. A good plan to follow is to start with the upper right third molar region and include all teeth of the upper arch, ending with the upper left third molar. The lower exposures

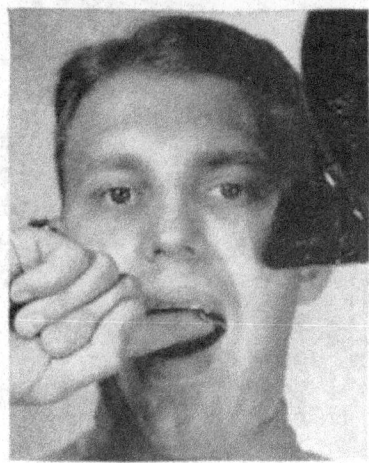

① Position.

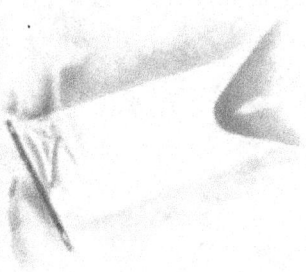

② Diagram of relation of rays to film. Tube inclined 30° above horizontal for average case.

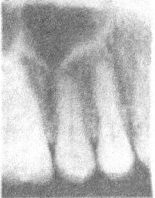

③ Resulting roentgenogram.

FIGURE 92.—Maxillary bicuspid area.

are started with the left molar area and include all teeth in the lower arch, ending with the lower right molar region.

111. Maxillary molar.—Adjust the head so the occlusal surfaces of the maxillary teeth are horizontal and the median plane of the face is vertical. Place the film packet in the mouth so that the long axis is horizontal and the anterior border of the film is at the middle of the second bicuspid, the lower border of the packet parallel to and slightly below the occlusal surfaces of the molars. The patient's index finger of the hand from the opposite side, other fingers closed, is placed

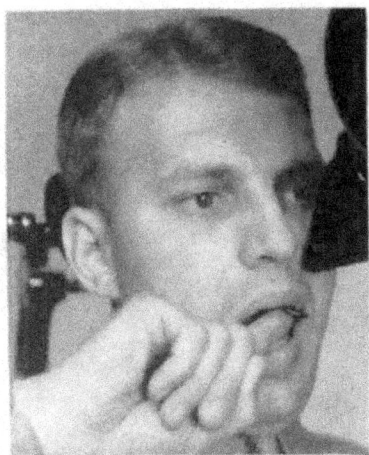

① Position.

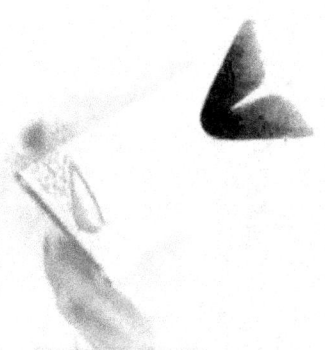

② Diagram of relation of rays to film. Tube inclined 45° above horizontal for average case.

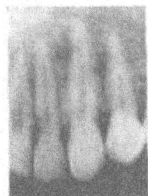

③ Resulting roentgenogram.

FIGURE 93.—Maxillary canine area.

against the surface of the packet holding it in contact with the crowns of the teeth and adjacent tissues. The film packet should not be bent and only sufficient pressure applied to stabilize the film during exposure. The tube is inclined to an average angle of 20° above the occlusal plane and the rays directed slightly distally, perpendicularly to the bisecting plane, through the second molar tooth and straight through the interproximal spaces (fig. 91). Maxillary impacted or malposed teeth may require special positioning of the film packet to give a satisfactory view. For exposure time see chart.

112. Maxillary bicuspid.—Place the film packet in the mouth so that the long axis is vertical, the anterior border of the film at the

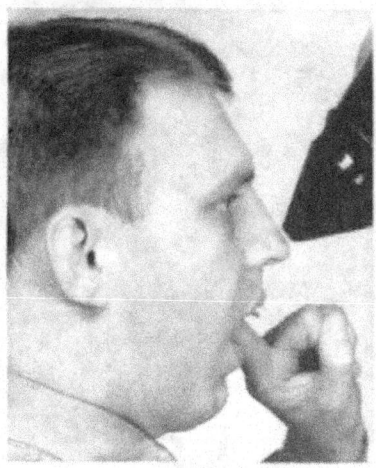

① Position.

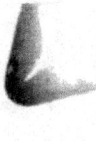

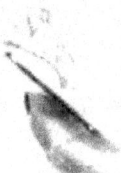

② Diagram of relation of rays to film. Tube inclined 40° above horizontal for average case.

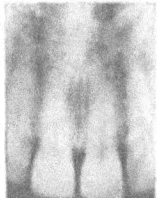

③ Resulting roentgenogram.

FIGURE 94.—Maxillary central incisor area.

middle of the canine, the lower border parallel to and slightly below the occlusal surfaces of the bicuspids. The tube is inclined to an average angle of 30° above the occlusal plane and the rays directed slightly distally, perpendicularly to the bisecting plane, straight through the apical thirds of the roots of the bicuspid teeth (fig. 92). For exposure time see chart.

113. Maxillary canine.—Place the film packet in the mouth with the long axis vertical and the lower border of the film parallel to and slightly below the incisal edges of the lateral and canine teeth. The anterior border bisects the central incisor on the same side with the canine opposite center of packet (do not bend the film). The

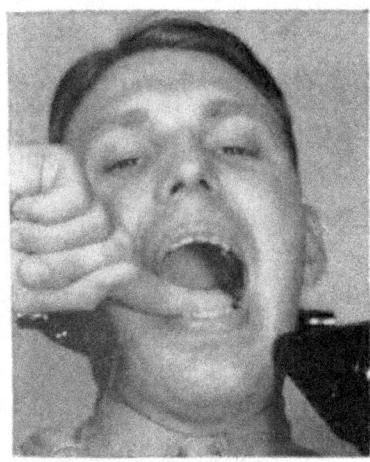

① Position.

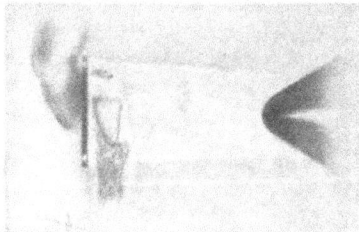

② Diagram of relation of rays to film. Tube inclined 5° below horizontal.

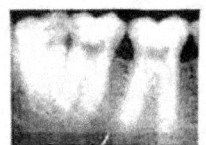

③ Resulting roentgenogram.

FIGURE 95.—Mandibular molar area.

tube is inclined to an average angle of 45° above the occlusal plane and rays directed through the apical third of the root of the canine tooth, perpendicularly to the bisecting plane, and straight through the interproximal spaces (fig. 93).

114. Maxillary incisor.—Place the film packet in the mouth with the long axis vertical, the center of the film on the median line of the upper arch, the lower border of the packet parallel to and slightly below the incisal edges of the incisors (do not bend the film). The tube is inclined to an average angle of 40° above the occlusal plane and the rays directed straight through between the apical thirds of the roots of the centrals, perpendicularly to the bisecting plane (fig. 94).

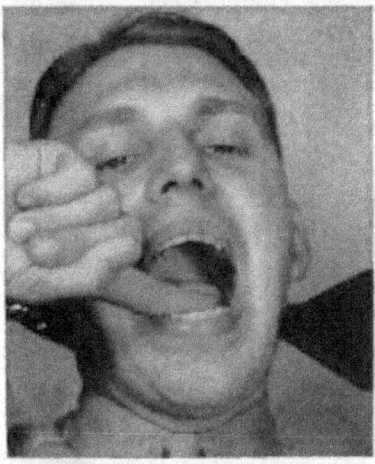

① Position.

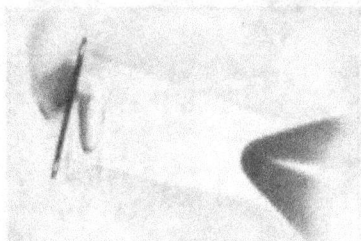

② Diagram of relation of rays to film. Tube inclined 10° below horizontal.

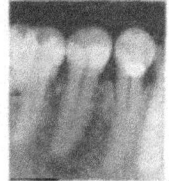

③ Resulting roentgenogram

FIGURE 96.—Mandibular bicuspid area.

115. Mandibular molar.—Place the patient's head so that the occlusal plane of the mandibular teeth is horizontal and the median plane of the face is vertical. Place the packet in the mouth with the long axis horizontal and the upper border of the film parallel to and slightly above the occlusal surfaces of the molars. It is placed alongside the tongue and far enough distally so that the third molar area will be included, anterior edge at middle of the second bicuspid. Mandibular impacted or malposed teeth may require special positioning of the film packet to give a satisfactory view. The patient's index finger of the hand from the opposite side, other fingers closed, is placed against the surface of the packet, holding it in contact with the crowns of the teeth and adjacent tissues. The packet should not be bent and only sufficient pressure applied to stabilize the film during exposure. The tube is inclined to an average angle of 5° below the occlusal plane and the rays directed through the roots of the second molars, perpendicularly to the bisecting plane, and straight through the interproximal spaces (fig. 95).

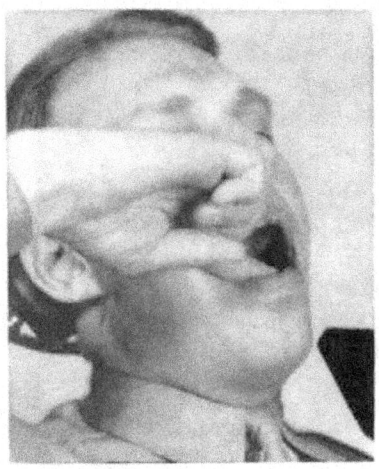

① Position.

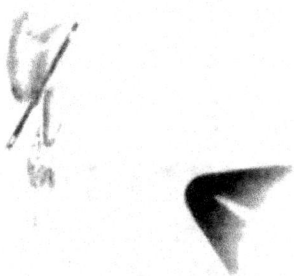

② Diagram of relation of rays to film. Tube inclined 20° below horizontal.

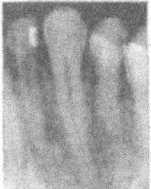

③ Resulting roentgenogram.

FIGURE 97.—Mandibular canine area.

116. Mandibular bicuspid.—Place the film packet in the mouth with the long axis vertical and the upper border of the film parallel to and slightly above the occlusal surfaces of the bicuspids. The anterior border should be about the middle of the canine. The tube is inclined to an average angle of 10° below the occlusal plane and the rays directed between the apical thirds of the roots of the bicuspid teeth, perpendicularly to the bisecting plane, and straight through the interproximal spaces (fig. 96). For exposure time see chart.

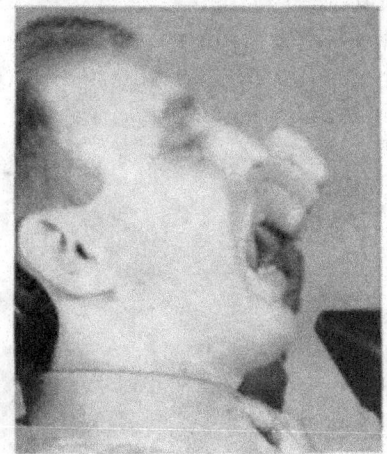

① Position.

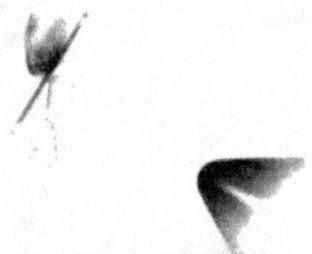

② Diagram of relation of rays to film. Tube inclined 15° below horizontal.

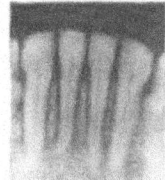

③ Resulting roentgenogram.

FIGURE 98.—Mandibular incisor area.

117. Mandibular canine.—Place the packet in the mouth with the long axis vertical and the upper border of the film parallel to and slightly above the incisal edges of the lateral and canine teeth. The anterior border of the film should be about the distal surface of the opposite central incisor, canine opposite the center of packet. The tube is inclined to an average angle of 20° below the occlusal plane and the rays directed through the apical third of the root of the canine tooth, perpendicularly to the bisecting plane, and straight through the interproximal spaces (fig. 97). For exposure time see chart.

118. **Mandibular incisor.**—Place the film packet in the mouth with the long axis vertical and the upper border parallel to and slightly above the incisal edges of the incisor teeth, the center of the film on the median line of the lower arch. The patient's index finger of either hand is placed against the center of the film with just enough pressure to hold it in place without bending it. The tube is inclined to an average angle of 15° below the occlusal plane and the rays directed between the apical thirds of the roots of the centrals.

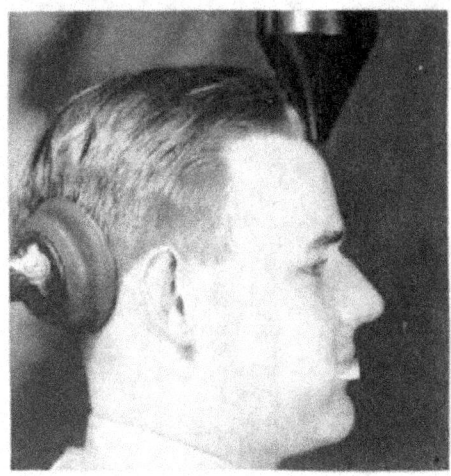

① Position of head, film, and tube.

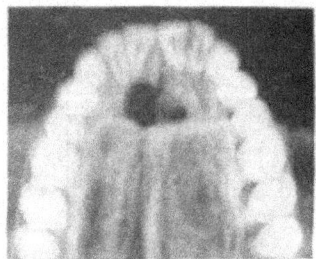

② Occlusal roentgenogram.

FIGURE 99.—Maxillary occlusal area (full view).

perpendicularly to the bisecting plane, and straight through the interproximal spaces (fig. 98).

119. **Occlusal examination.**—A third type of intra-oral examination is the occlusal film. In no way should it be substituted for the other types but it does have a very great value in certain situations. It assists in locating fractures, residual roots, impacted teeth, foreign bodies, cysts, sialolithiasis (stones), etc. It also can be used

to advantage in cases of trismus where it is impossible for the patient to open the mouth sufficiently to use standard films. Occlusal films are supplied in lead-backed packets similar to the standard dental films, but measuring 2¼ by 3 inches.

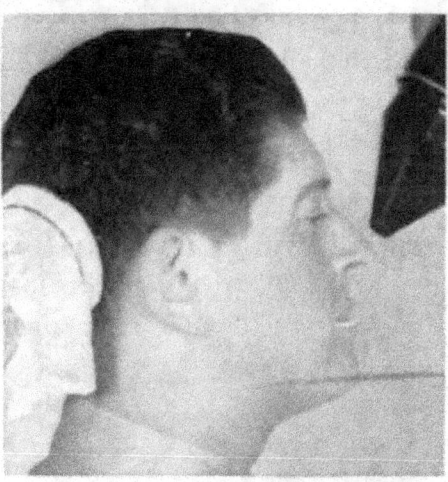

① Position of head, film, and tube.

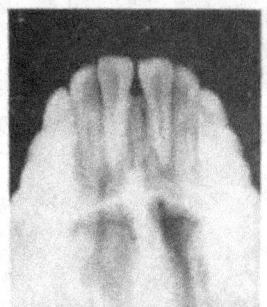

② Occlusal roentgenogram.

FIGURE 100.—Maxillary central and lateral incisor areas (occlusal view).

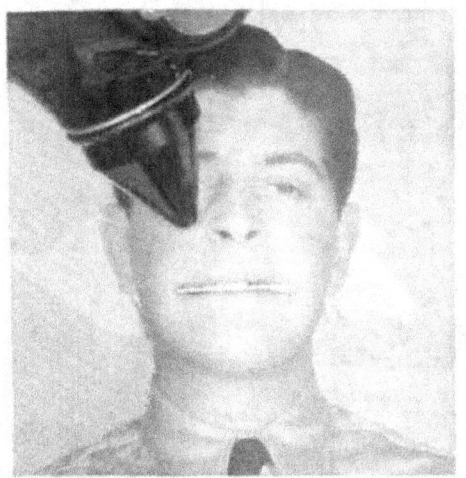 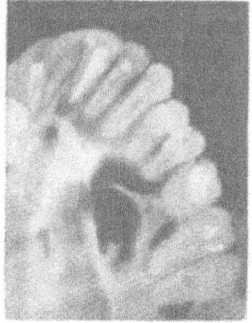

① Position for occlusal film.   ② Occlusal roentgenogram.

FIGURE 101.—Maxillary canine, bicuspid, and molar areas (occlusal view).

120. Maxillary occlusal (full view).—Adjust the head so that the occlusal surfaces of the maxillary teeth are horizontal; median line of face vertical. The film packet is placed in the mouth with either the short axis or long axis at right angle to median line of face. The teeth are closed gently but firmly against the film packet. The tube is adjusted so that the point of the cone touches the top of the forehead in the median line and the rays are directed downward, perpendicularly to the plane of the packet (fig. 99). For exposure time see chart.

121. Maxillary central and lateral incisor.—The tube is inclined to an average angle of 65° above the occlusal plane, centering the cone slightly above the tip of the nose in the median line, directing

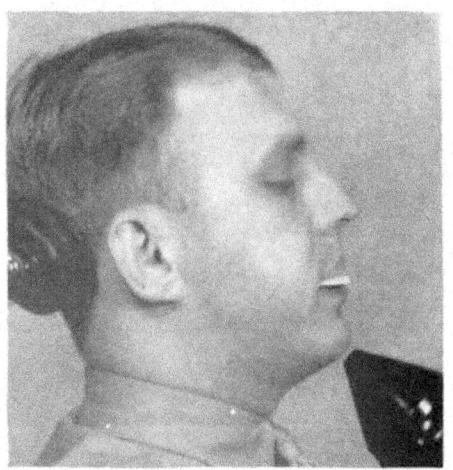

① Position of head, film, and tube.

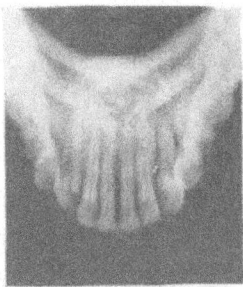

② Occlusal roentgenogram.

FIGURE 102.—Mandibular central and lateral incisor areas (occlusal view).

the rays downward and distally through the nose and apical thirds of the roots of the maxillary central incisors toward the plane of the packet (fig. 100). For exposure time see chart.

122. Maxillary canine, bicuspid, and molar.—The tube is inclined to an average angle of 60° above the occlusal plane and the cone centered on the canine fossa, directing the rays through the periapical region of the canine and first bicuspid toward the plane of the packet (fig. 101). For exposure time see chart.

123. Mandibular central and lateral incisor.—The patient's head is tilted backward so that the occlusal plane of the teeth is 55°

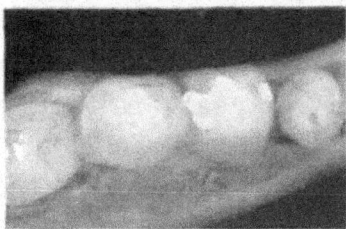

NOTE.—This is same position and technique as illustrated in figure 104 except that small dental film was used.

FIGURE 103.—Occlusal roentgenogram of mandibular molar area on standard dental film.

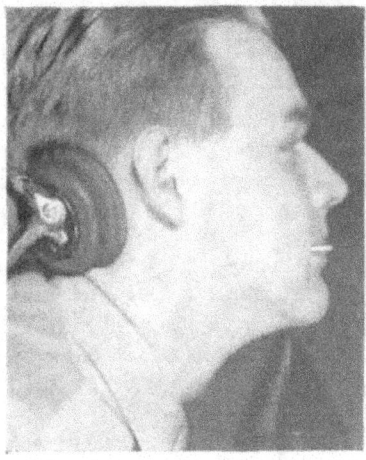

① Position for occlusal film.

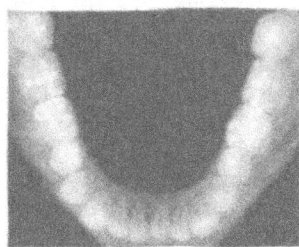

② Occlusal roentgenogram on occlusal film (for same technique using dental film, see fig. 103).

FIGURE 104.—Mandibular area (full view).

above horizontal. The median line of the face is vertical. The packet is placed in the mouth with either the long or short axis at right angles to the median line of the face. The teeth are closed gently but firmly against the film packet. The tube is horizontal and the cone centered on the point of the chin, directing the rays through the apical thirds of the mandibular central incisors (fig. 102).

124. Mandibular canine, bicuspid, and molar.—Adjust the head so that the occlusal plane is perpendicular to the horizontal plane and place packet in the mouth parallel to the mandibular occlusal plane. The tube is horizontal and cone centered on the lower border of the mandible below the first molar, directing the rays toward the plane of the film (fig. 103). For exposure time see chart.

125. Mandibular occlusal (full view).—Adjust the head so that the occlusal plane is perpendicular to the horizontal plane and place packet in the mouth parallel to the mandibular occlusal plane. The tube is horizontal and the cone is centered in the median line, directing the rays perpendicularly toward the packet (fig. 104). For edentulous cases cotton rolls may be used to assist in the retention of the film in the mouth. For exposure time see chart.

EXPOSURE TIME CHART

Area	Average degree of angulation	Regular film			Radiatized film			Extra-fast film		
		Small-sized face	Medium-sized face	Large-sized face	Small-sized face	Medium-sized face	Large-sized face	Small-sized face	Medium-sized face	Large-sized face
		Seconds	Seconds	Seconds	Seconds	Seconds	Seconds	Seconds	Seconds	Seconds
Maxillary—										
Molar	+20	7	8	9	3½	4	4½	2	2¼	2½
Bicuspid	+30	3	4	5	2	2½	3	1	1¼	1½
Cuspid	+45	4	5	6	2½	3	3½	1¼	1½	1¾
Central	+40	4	5	6	2½	3	3½	1¼	1½	1¾
Mandibular—										
Molar	−5	4	5	6	2½	3	3½	1¼	1½	1¾
Bicuspid	−10	3	4	5	2	2½	3	1	1¼	1½
Cuspid	−20	3	4	5	2	2½	3	1	1¼	1½
Incisor	−15	3	4	5	2	2¼	2½	1	1¼	1½

NOTE.—For edentulous mouths increase degree of angulation from 5° to 10° and shorten above exposure time by 25 percent.

Section III

EXTRA-ORAL ROENTGENOGRAPHY

	Paragraph
General	126
Body of mandible and ramus	127
Temporomandibular articulation	128
Bones of face	129

126. General.—The second type of dental X-ray examination is extra-oral roentgenography. It is, as the term applies, a roentgenogram taken with the film outside the mouth. The intra-oral method of taking roentgenograms of the teeth is the one usually followed to diagnose conditions involving small areas such as abscesses, root canal fillings, caries, etc. Such films are desirable as they give more contrast and detail than extra-oral films, since they are taken in much closer relation to the object and have less superimposition of shadows. But frequently this type of roentgenogram leaves some doubt or only shows part of the area involved. In cases of this type, extra-oral roentgenograms should be taken to give a more complete view of the region involved. It is also indicated in locating fractures, impacted teeth, cysts, etc.

a. Extra-oral roentgenography includes X-ray examination of—

(1) Body of mandible.
(2) Angle of mandible.
(3) Ramus of mandible.
(4) Temporomandibular articulation.
(5) Bones of face.

b. For extra-oral X-rays larger films are necessary. Pictures of the maxillae and mandible and other facial bones are usually made on 8- by 10-inch films. Full skull pictures require 10- by 14-inch size. These films are packed, 12 in a box, and wrapped in black paper with a separate sheet folded over each film, separating them from each other. Cassettes or paper film holders should be loaded in the darkroom and unused films kept in a box to protect them from exposure to light.

c. The technique described in the following paragraphs has been found to be very satisfactory, requiring only three films to give a good view of the mandible and other facial bones, one film for lateral view of the temporomandibular articulation. These may be made stereoscopically or angulation modified to improve the view of certain areas. The same technique can also be employed on litter cases or bed patients which is a distinct advantage in roentgenographing sick or seriously wounded patients.

127. Body of mandible and ramus.—Have the patient sit erect in the chair, head forward (headrest supporting it), median-line plane vertical, shoulders back, chin up so that the lower border of the mandible is parallel to the floor (fig. 105). By keeping the head well forward and chin up, the cervical vertebrae are kept from overshadowing the condyloid process and ramus. In case of bed patients or litter cases the chin is elevated and head raised so that the lower border of the mandible will be parallel to the walls. Adjust the head of the machine so that the cone is about 4 inches from the skin and points under the angle and body of one side of the mandible, using the alveolar process region of the third molar tooth of the opposite side as the center of the field. Further adjust the angle of

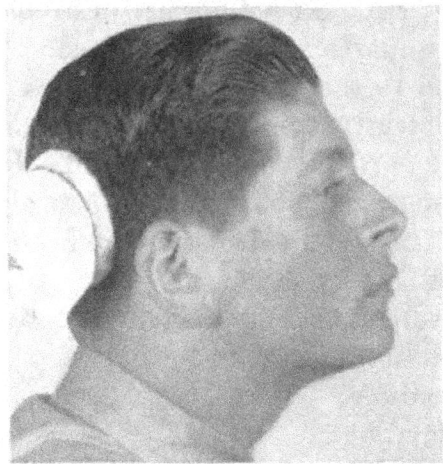

NOTE.—Headrest is adjusted in forward position so that patient sits erect with chin up and head well forward (lower border of mandible parallel to floor).

FIGURE 105.—Position of head for lateral extra-oral roentgenography of mandible.

the cone so that rays from the target can pass under the near side of angle of mandible and expose the condyloid head of the opposite side. This gives an angle from the horizontal of 15° to 20°. If the cassette is held so that the center rays from the target are perpendicular to it, an angle is formed between the plane of the film and plane of the long axis of the ramus (verticle angle) (fig. 106①). Bisect this angle and move the cassette into the new position. Another angle is now formed by the plane of the film and the long axis of the body of the mandible (horizontal angle) (fig. 106②). Bisect this angle and move the anterior edge of the cassette into the new position (fig. 106③ and 107①). This exposure will project an image of the body and ramus of the mandible on the film with the length of each approximately correct (fig. 107②).

128. Temporomandibular articulation.

—Palpate the sigmoid notch of the opposite side to be exposed and have patient open the mouth to move the condyles forward (about 3 centimeters between anterior teeth). Remove the cone and adjust the head of the machine

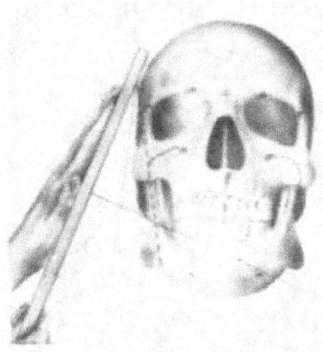

① Vertical angle formed between plane of cassette and plane of long axis of ramus.

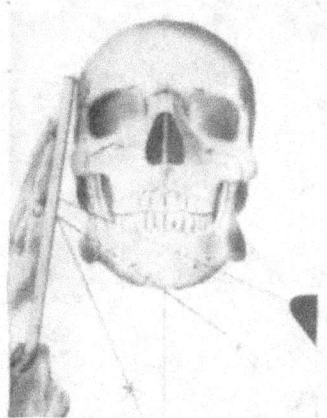

② Cassette moved to bisect vertical angle. Horizontal angle between plane of cassette and long axis of body of mandible is now indicated in sketch.

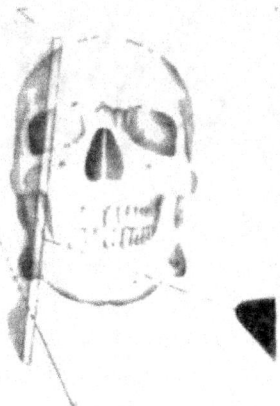

③ Keeping vertical plane of cassette constant, forward edge is now moved so that horizontal plane is bisected (this is correct position).

FIGURE 106.

so that the target will be close to the space above the sigmoid notch and under the zygomatic arch, so that the rays can pass directly through toward the articulation of the opposite side. The film is held perpendicular to these rays and the exposure made (fig. 108). Due to the short target film distance, the images are slightly enlarged and the condyloid head is shown with little or no superimposed shadows.

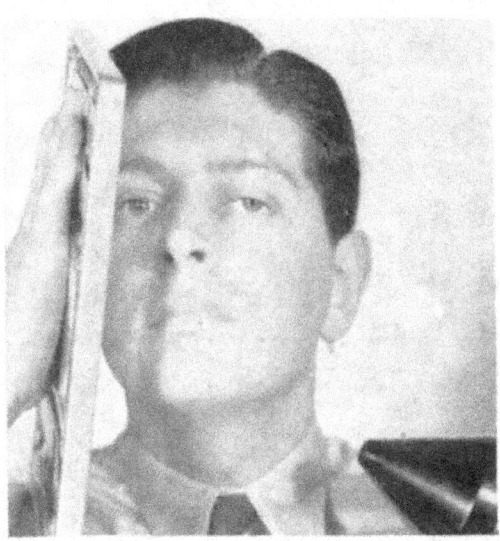

① Position of head, cassette, and tube for correct image of body and ramus of mandible (same as fig. 106③).

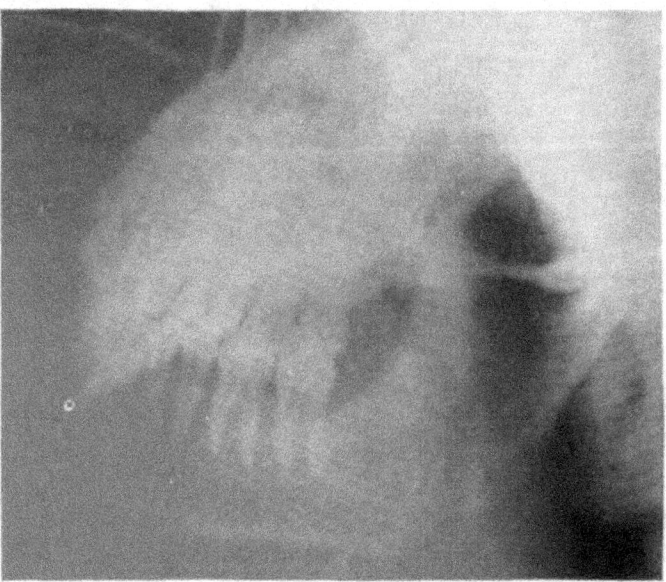

② Resulting roentgenogram of body and ramus of mandible.
FIGURE 107.

129. Bones of face.—Lower the arm of the dental chair and place the cassette on the seat, using this as an adjustable table for exposure. Have patient sit on an ordinary chair facing the side of the dental

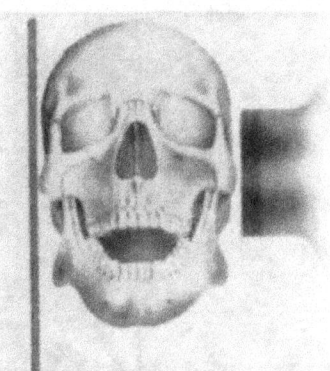

① Diagram of relation of head, tube (cone removed), and film for roentgenography of temporomandibular articulation.

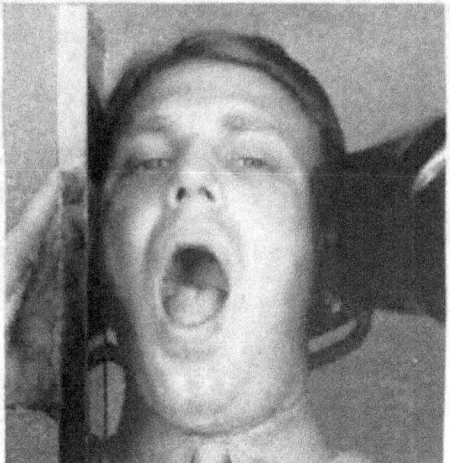

② Photograph of this position.

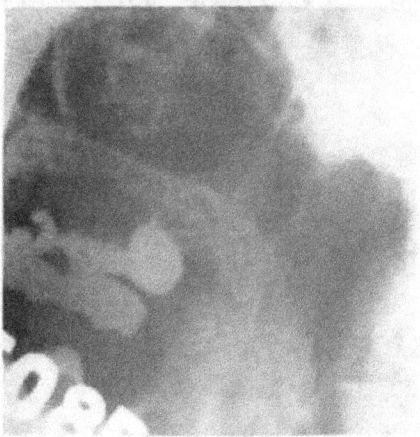

③ Resulting roentgenogram of temporomandibular articulation.

FIGURE 108.

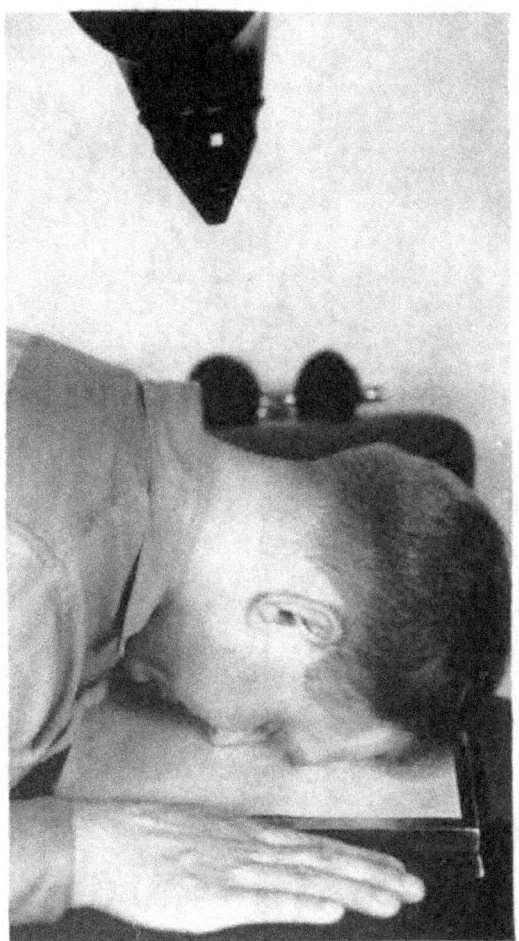

① Position for antero-posterior view of bones of face.

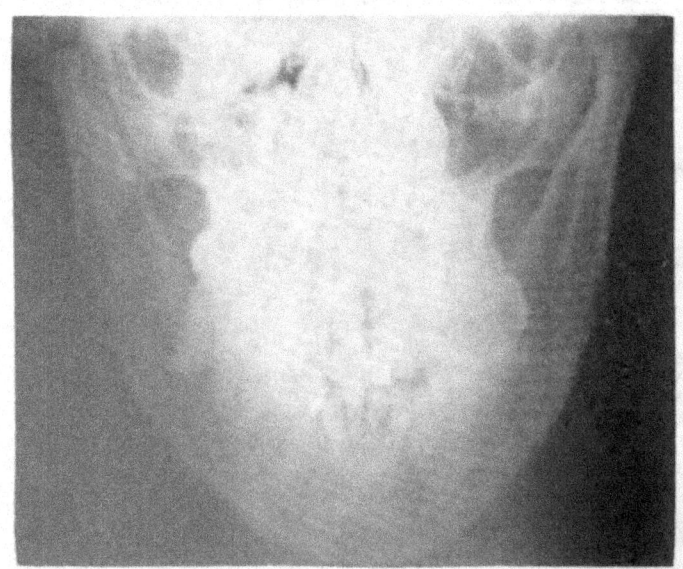

② Roentgenogram of bones of face.

FIGURE 109.

chair, close enough to lean over the cassette, one hand on either side to steady the position; place forehead and nose on the cassette so that the mandible and facial bones can be projected on the film. A target film distance of 24 inches is used and rays directed in the median-line plane between the condyloid processes of the mandible, forming about a 10° angle from the perpendicular toward the patient's shoulders. This gets the rays through under the occipital portion of the skull (fig. 109).

Section IV

PROCESSING OF X-RAY FILMS

	Paragraph
General	130
Darkroom	131
Illumination	132
Processing tank	133
Thermometer	134
Clock	135
Film holders	136
Processing solutions	137
Technique of processing films by time-temperature chart	138

130. General.—Precise methods in the developing of X-ray films are just as essential in attaining good results as the utilization of precise exposure technique. If the correct procedure is followed throughout, the resulting roentgenogram will leave nothing to be desired and the technician can perform his work with every assurance that he is providing roentgenograms of the maximum quality. If, on the other hand, the processing procedure is carelessly done and directions not carefully followed, all the care that was exercised during the exposure of the films will be time lost. The method to be followed is known as the standardized time-temperature processing procedure.

131. Darkroom.—As the films used in X-ray work are very sensitive to light, much more so than ordinary photographic films, it is important to have a good darkroom. It need not be such a large room, but it must be constructed so that no light could enter through cracks or crevices. In addition, the door should have an inside lock so that no one could accidentally open it or enter while films are being processed. A better type of construction plan would be to have a maze for entering the darkroom provided with enough turns to keep out light. The walls should be painted black and the ceiling may be white, which will reflect sufficient illumination when the correct type of safelight is used. The room should be supplied with both hot and cold water and the pipes should lead to a mixing valve so that the temperature of the flow can be regulated. Adequate ventilation must not be overlooked and the use of some forced change of air employing a ventilator fan is advisable.

132. Illumination.—For the illumination of the darkroom a light that is photographically safe must be used. There are numerous kinds of these lights available, but the standard for a safelight is as follows: It must be possible to permit undeveloped films to be exposed to the light at a distance of 3 feet for a period of 1 minute without the least evidence of fogging.

133. Processing tank.—A suitable tank for processing films is an important part of the darkroom equipment. The tank should be constructed of corrosion-resistant material such as porcelain, hard rubber, or certain rust-resistant metals. Compartments or divisions are provided for the developing and fixing solutions with a larger section for water. A connection with a mixing valve, hot or cold water, for temperature control is desirable, thereby eliminating guesswork.

134. Thermometer.—As it is essential to process the film at the predetermined temperature, the tank must be equipped with a thermometer that will register the exact temperature of the circulating water.

135. Clock.—Because of the direct relationship between temperature and time in the processing procedure, it is necessary to know the exact time that any given film is to be left in each solution. For this purpose a good watch will serve, but it is much better to use an interval timer. This gives the time in minutes and fractions of minutes and is equipped with an alarm which sounds to indicate the expiration of the time interval selected.

136. Film holders.—There are two types of film holders. For the small intra-oral films, clip holders; for the larger extra-oral films, frame holders (fig. 110).

137. Processing solutions.—The chemicals for developing and fixing are put in moistureproof containers and in the proper proportions, ready to mix with water. They come in sizes which will make 5 gallons of solution. The developing solution and the fixing solution are each prepared according to manufacturer's instructions on the package.

a. Frequently the processing chemicals are not obtainable in the ready-to-mix form. Therefore it is necessary for the X-ray technician to know the formula of a developer and a fixing solution and the method of making each from their component parts. The following formulas are for making 6 gallons of each solution, but may

DENTAL TECHNICIANS

TM 8-225
137

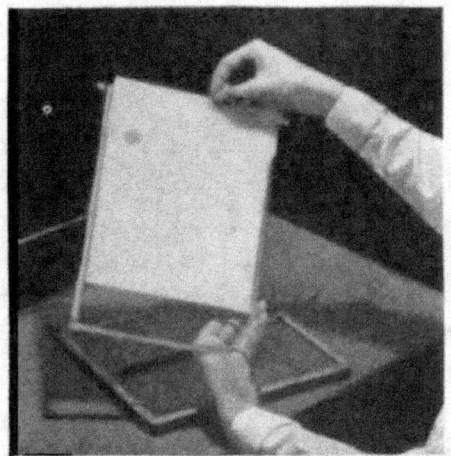

① Intra-oral.   ② Extra-oral.

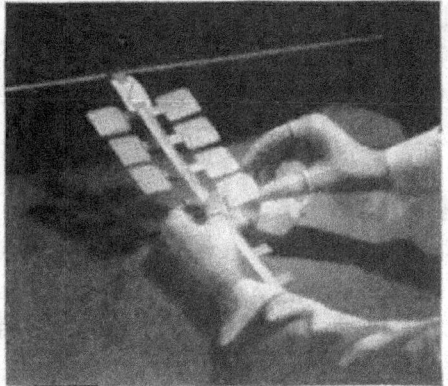

FIGURE 110.—Placing film on developing hanger.

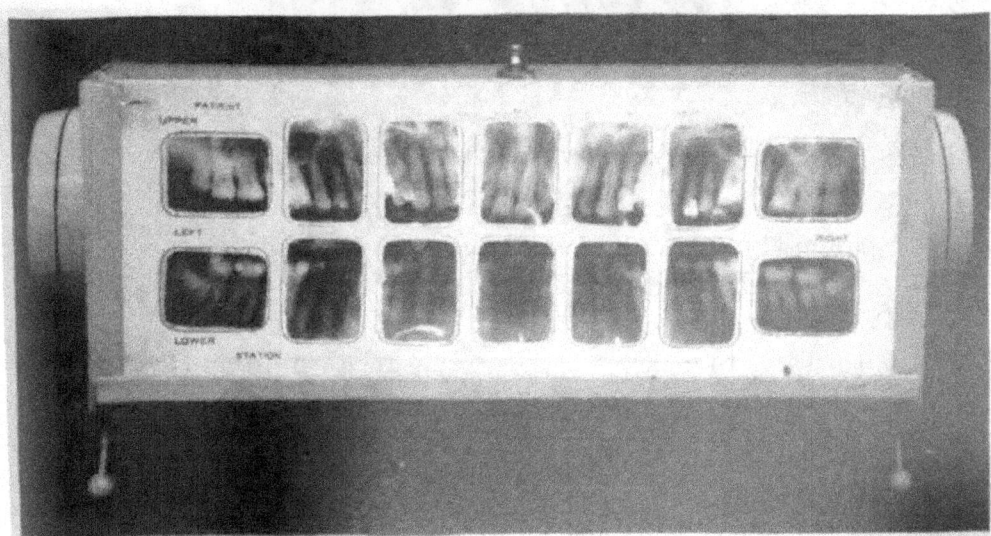

FIGURE 111.—Dental films in standard mount.

TM 8-225
137   MEDICAL DEPARTMENT

be cut down by the technician to apply to any amount that may be necessary.

(1) *Formula for developer.*

Elon	60 grams.
Sodium sulfite	2,500 grams.
Hydroquinone	240 grams.
Sodium carbonate	1,250 grams (desiccated).
Potassium bromide	150 grams.
Cold water to make	24 liters (6 gallons).

(*a*) Weigh out the individual chemicals on small pieces of paper. Mix in white enameled containers.

(*b*) Dissolve them individually in as small a volume of warm water as possible (125° F.).

(*c*) Mix a handful of dry sulfite with the elon and hydroquinone before dissolving them.

(*d*) Pour the solutions of elon and hydroquinone together.

(*e*) Pour the solutions of sodium sulfite and sodium carbonate together.

(*f*) Add the potassium bromide solution to the solution just mixed.

(*g*) Add the elon and hydroquinone mixture to the mixture of soda and bromide solutions.

(*h*) Add cold water to make the necessary volume.

(*i*) Filter each solution before mixing through six thicknesses of gauze.

(2) *Formula for fixing bath (hypo).*

Sodium thiosulfate (hypo)	66 kilograms.
Water to make	16 liters.

When fully dissolved add following hardening solution:

Water	4 liters.
Sodium sulfite	300 grams.
Acetic acid (glacial)	260 cubic centimeters.
Potassium alum (granular)	300 grams.
Cold water to make	8 liters (total 24 liters (6 gal.)).

(*a*) Dissolve the chemicals in water at about 125° F. in the order given.

(*b*) The sodium sulfite must be completely dissolved before adding the acetic acid.

(*c*) Add the alum to the sulfite-acid solution and stir until a clear solution appears.

(*d*) When this clear sulfite-acid-alum solution has cooled, add it slowly, stirring constantly, to the cool and thoroughly dissolved hypo solution.

(*e*) Filter through six thicknesses of gauze.

b. The developing solution is poured into one of the hard rubber tanks and the hypo solution in the other. It is most important to have these tanks absolutely clean before adding the solutions. They should also be equipped with a cover and the solutions kept covered when not in use. This prevents oxidation which is an important factor in solutions becoming inactive.

138. Technique of processing films by time-temperature chart.—All necessary equipment should have a definite place in the darkroom for when the lights are turned out and development begun, the technician will not be able to locate misplaced objects. The hands must be clean and dry, otherwise the films when finished will contain finger marks which cannot be removed.

a. Remove the lightproof wrapper from around the film.

b. Place the film on the film holder, holding the film lightly by the edges, avoiding touching the surface with the fingers as this will leave fingerprints and smudges.

c. Adjust the time interval clock for the developing time prescribed by the chart, or place a watch where the time can be noted.

d. The timing should start just as soon as the film is placed in the developing solution.

e. Place the film holder with the film attached in the tank containing the developing solution. Make certain that the film does not touch the side of the tank or other films. The emulsion will adhere to either and will not develop properly at the contact point. This will leave a spot on the film having the appearance of a radiopaque area. Film holders that have not been thoroughly washed after they have been once immersed in hypo may also cause streaks. The dried hypo dissolves in the developing solution and runs over the emulsion of the film, dissolving the silver halide salts, causing streaks of underdevelopment.

f. When the prescribed developing time has elapsed for the film as given on the chart, it is removed and placed in circulating water for 30 seconds or longer to remove all traces of the solution. If this is not done the developer will be carried over into the fixing bath, neutralizing its acid content and contaminating it.

g. The films are placed in the hypo or fixing bath and should remain there for twice the time required to remove these salts. Under no circumstances should they be taken out of the solution until they are clear, 8 to 10 minutes being advisable. The purpose of fixation is to remove all unexposed silver salts from the emulsion, permanently fix the image brought up by the developer, and harden the emulsion.

h. Upon completion of fixation the films should be immersed in circulating water, 65° F., and washed for 30 minutes to assure the complete removal of the fixing bath from the emulsion. This is a most important step in the processing because the radiograph will in time turn yellow and fade if any chemicals of the fixing bath remain in the solution.

i. Drying is the last step in processing. Quick drying can be accomplished by placing the film in a dryer, a box-shaped cabinet with a heating element at one end and an electric suction fan at the other. The flow of warm air over the films suspended on the hangars in the cabinet hastens drying. Films can also be dried in the open air and somewhat hastened by having a fan so placed that the air is kept circulating around them.

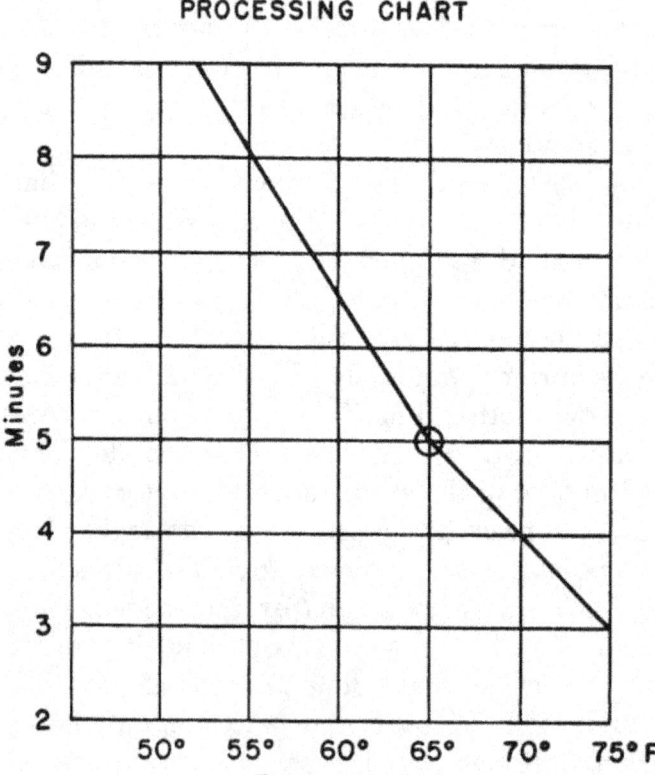

PROCESSING CHART

Chapter 5

DENTAL HYGIENIST

	Paragraphs
Section I. General	139
II. Structure and physiology	140–142
III. Dental caries	143–144
IV. Other diseases of mouth	145–153
V. Saliva, deposits, and accretions upon teeth	154–157
VI. Technique of dental prophylaxis	158–161
VII. System for instrumentation and polishing	162–165
VIII. Instructions to patient	166–167
IX. Preparations for mouth and teeth	168–170

Section I

GENERAL

	Paragraph
Definitions	139

139. Definitions.—Dental hygiene is the science of the health of the teeth and their surrounding tissues. It is maintained by dental prophylaxis and daily home care of the mouth. Dental prophylaxis is that scientific effort either operative, educational, or therapeutic which tends to prevent diseases of the teeth and their surrounding tissues. The dental hygienist has been developed as a co-worker in dentistry to assist in securing clean mouths, sound teeth, and healthy gums for the patients by dental prophylaxis and education.

Section II

STRUCTURE AND PHYSIOLOGY

	Paragraph
Structure of teeth	140
Occlusion	141
Mastication	142

140. Structure of teeth.—A tooth is divided into two parts, the crown and the root. The crown is that portion which projects above the gum; the root is that portion which normally is surrounded by gum and alveolar process. The bulk of the tooth is composed of dentine which gives it shape and incloses the pulp cavity. The crown portion of the dentine is covered by cementum which slightly overlaps the enamel at the gingival margin. The pulp cavity is in the center of the tooth extending the whole length of the root and into the crown.

Within the pulp cavity is located the tooth pulp, a soft, highly sensitive, vascular organ, commonly but incorrectly called the nerve. The pulp cavity is divided into two parts, that in the crown is known as the pulp chamber, and that in the root is known as the root canal. The root canal communicates with the exterior through one or more openings at the end of the root known as apical foramina through which pass the nerve and blood vessels of the tooth. Surrounding the

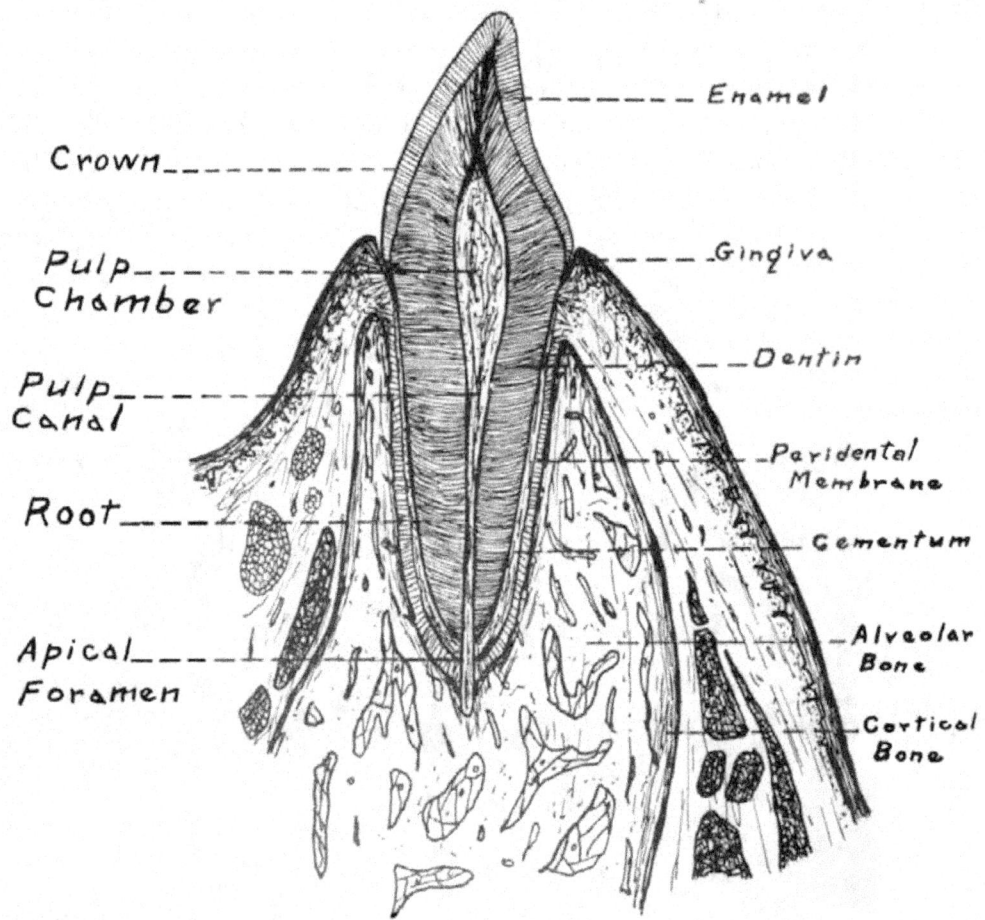

FIGURE 112.—Cross-section diagram showing various tissues which make up tooth, bone, and gingiva.

root and separating it from the bony socket is a fibrous tissue known as peridental membrane which binds the tooth to the supporting bone. Covering the bony process (alveolar process) is a dense fibrous connective tissue covered with epithelium which we call the gingiva or gum (fig. 112).

141. Occlusion.—The teeth are arranged in two curving arches, the lower of which is somewhat smaller so that the upper overlaps it. The teeth of one arch do not meet those of the other in an end to end arrangement but cusps of the lower are dovetailed with the cusps of

the upper. It is the sliding together of these various cusps in a scissorlike action that properly prepares the food for digestion. Normal arrangement of the arches when the jaws are closed is known as occlusion. Any deviation of the teeth or arches from the normal relationship is termed malocclusion.

142. Mastication.—*a.* Mastication is a voluntary act which is continued reflexly and automatically by the muscles active in moving the mandible. These may be divided into two sets: muscles of mastication which bring the lower teeth in contact with the upper in the process of chewing by raising the mandible; and depressor muscles or those which pull the mandible downward as in opening the mouth.

(1) The muscles of mastication are—
- Temporal.
- Masseter.
- Buccinator.
- Internal pterygoid.
- External pterygoid.

(2) The depressor muscles are—
- Geniohyoid.
- Mylohyoid.
- Digastric.
- Platysma.

b. The chief muscles of the tongue are the genioglossus and the styloglossus. Their action is to thrust the tongue forward, retract, and depress it. Working in balanced harmony with the muscles that move the mandible and those that move the tongue are the muscles of expression. They are found in the lips and cheeks and produce many varied facial expressions.

c. During the process of mastication, saliva is poured in large quantities into the mouth. The secretion of saliva is the result of reflex stimulation of the nerves supplying the salivary glands. The nerves are stimulated by the movements of mastication and the taste and smell of food.

Section III

DENTAL CARIES

	Paragraph
General	143
Theory of cause	144

143. General.—Dental caries (tooth decay) is a destructive process affecting the hard dental tissues, the enamel, dentine, and cementum. Dental caries always has its inception upon the external or exposed surface of a tooth and travels toward the pulp. Certain surfaces of the teeth are more susceptible to tooth decay than others. In general those surfaces of the teeth that are subjected to the cleansing action of the tongue, lips, and cheeks or those tooth surfaces which are kept clean by the friction of tough or fibrous foods are less likely to decay. Locations where food particles can find an undisturbed lodgment such as natural pits and depressions in the masticating surfaces of the molars and bicuspids, sulci between the cusps, and especially the approximating surfaces of the teeth are very susceptible to the carious process.

144. Theory of cause.—The most generally accepted theory for the cause of dental caries is that of Dr. W. D. Miller, who, through his extensive research, demonstrated that dental caries is produced by bacterial fermentation of carbohydrate food debris about the teeth which results in decalcification of the inorganic material of the teeth by the acids so formed, with a simultaneous invasion and destruction of the organic material of the teeth. It is known from experience that teeth decay more rapidly in early life than in adult life, that some individuals are markedly more susceptible to decay than others, and that some individuals with extremely filthy mouths are immune to caries. These facts can only be explained by assigning another factor to the cause of dental decay which must in some way be concerned with the general health of the individual. This factor, because it is connected with the general health and because it must act before the local cause of the decay does, is referred to as a predisposing factor or a systemic factor. About this predisposing factor very little is known and authorities have variously attributed it to faulty diet, imperfections in the calcified tooth structure, endocrine gland disturbances, and various other causes. However, it is generally agreed that teeth decay more readily in a filthy mouth and that if proper hygiene is maintained tooth decay may be controlled.

Section IV

OTHER DISEASES OF MOUTH

	Paragraph
Periodontal diseases	145
Periodontoclasia	146
Causes of periodontoclasia	147
Vincent's stomatitis	148
Stomatitis apthous	149
Bismuth stomatitis	150
Gingivitis	151
Hypertrophic gingivitis	152
Atrophy or recession of gingivae or gums	153

145. Periodontal diseases.—A number of diseases affect the tissues immediately surrounding the tooth root. These diseases involve first the gum tissue (gingiva), then the periodontal membrane, and finally involve the bone. The dental diseases of this group are called periodontal diseases.

146. Periodontoclasia.—Periodontoclasia (paradentosis) is the most common of the periodontal diseases. It produces a progressive destruction of the supporting tissues of the teeth until after many years the teeth become so loose that they must be extracted. There is more than one type of periodontoclasia; however, this manual will not deal with the different types. Generally, periodontoclasia begins with an inflammation of the tissues around the necks of the teeth. This inflammation of the gingival tissues is called a gingivitis. If not treated, generally the gingivitis progresses to the deeper tissues and the disease is established. Periodontoclasia is a very slowly progressing disease which becomes chronic and is difficult to cure. As the disease progresses, the tissue nearest the tooth root is destroyed and a pocket is formed. As these pockets around the teeth become deeper, the teeth loosen and finally must be extracted.

147. Causes of periodontoclasia.—These may be divided into two groups: systemic and local.

a. The systemic causes of periodontoclasia are not fully understood but they exist because patients with some systemic diseases, such as diabetes or certain diseases of the thyroid gland, are definitely more susceptible to periodontoclasia. Also, improvement in the general health by proper diet, rest, and elimination of other infectious conditions will improve the periodontoclasia.

b. The local causes of periodontoclasia include any factor which chronically irritates the gum margin, abnormal forces exerted over a long period of time on the tooth or teeth, and finally bacterial invasion of the tissues. The irritating factors are, in most cases, calcareous deposits on the teeth (calculus) and poorly finished dental restorations. The dental hygienist assists in the treatment of this disease by removing deposits on the teeth which are responsible for a large part of the irritation and by helping the patient to maintain a high degree of oral hygiene.

148. Vincent's stomatitis.—This disease is an acute infection of the mouth which is characterized by deep painful ulcers on the mucous membrane. The ulceration usually appears around the necks of the teeth but may appear on the cheeks, tongue, palate, or tonsils. The disease is characterized by pain, a gray membrane covering the ulcers and adjacent tissues, a foul odor, and acute inflammation of the involved tissues. This infection is contagious and may be transmitted from person to person by using a common drinking glass, passing a cigarette from one to another, kissing, or using another's eating utensils which had not been thoroughly washed. The treatment is the responsibility of the dentist.

149. Stomatitis apthous.—This appears as a yellowish-white, depressed, painful ulcer; sometimes there are more than one of these ulcers. They are commonly called canker sores.

150. Bismuth stomatitis.—This is caused by taking bismuth compounds, usually in the treatment of syphilis. It is characterized by sore and swollen gums and a metallic taste.

151. Gingivitis.—Gingivitis or inflammation of the gums may appear temporarily as a result of poor hygiene or it may be a precursor of periodontoclasia.

152. Hypertrophic gingivitis.—This is an inflammation of the gums characterized by marked swelling. This commonly appears as a response to some irritant either local or systemic. It appears in response to the ingestion of certain drugs and is commonly found in pregnant women as a reaction to their gestation.

153. Atrophy or recession of gingivae or gums.—This is another response of the gingival tissues to certain irritants. The tissues shrink away from the necks of the teeth, exposing part of the root. It generally accompanies old age and may appear in response to long continued irritation from some source such as abuse from improper use of the tooth brush.

Section V

SALIVA, DEPOSITS, AND ACCRETIONS UPON TEETH

	Paragraph
Saliva	154
Mucin plaques	155
Calculus	156
Green stain	157

154. Saliva.—Saliva is the fluid secretion found in the mouth and consists of a mixture of the secretions of the parotid gland, the submaxillary gland, the sublingual gland, and from innumerable mucous glands of the mucous membrane of the floor of the mouth, the palate, cheeks, and inner lining of the lips. Saliva consists of water, inorganic salts, some mucin, and an enzyme called ptyalin. It is normally colorless, odorless, and tasteless, and has a slightly alkaline reaction. Saliva has the following distinct functions:

a. By softening and moistening the food with mucin it lubricates it and insures smooth passage along the oesophagus.

b. By dissolving dry and solid food it provides a necessary step in the process of stimulating taste nerves, and taste sensations play an important part in the secretion of gastric fluid.

c. By virtue of the enzyme which it contains it changes starch to simple substances, that is, dextrin and maltose.

155. Mucin plaques.—Mucin plaques are precipitated upon the teeth by the action of weak acids and acid salts upon the mucin in the saliva. These acids usually are formed by the acid-forming action of certain bacteria on sugar. These plaques so formed are localized on all tooth surfaces that are unprotected by the friction of food in mastication, of tongue, or lips. The bacterial plaque is the essential factor in the localization of tooth decay and the most important characteristic cause. The bacterial plaque is soluble in a solution of three parts water and one part hydrogen peroxide. This solution may be used as a dentifrice by patients who are constitutionally susceptible to caries.

156. Calculus.—The precipitation of mucin by acids is the general factor which underlies the deposition of practically all deposits and accretions on the teeth. The earthy salts (phosphates and carbonates) that are held in the solution in the saliva by the escape of carbon dioxide combine and are precipitated within the substance of the mucin plaque to form a mass called calculus or tartar. Calculus varies in the rapidity with which it is formed, in its density, and in the tenacity with which it adheres to the tooth structure. Calculus which is formed rapidly and in large masses is usually soft. The hardness of calculus depends on the amount of its lime constituent in proportion to the mucin constituent. The hardest calculus is found just under the gum margin and is somewhat more difficult to remove than the soft type which is found on the crowns of the teeth. It occurs more abundantly near the orifices of the salivary ducts, and therefore is most often seen on the lingual surface of the lower incisors and the buccal surfaces of the upper molars. Calculus causes an inflammation of the gingival tissues, which is a factor in the cause of periodontoclasia. All deposits should be removed from the teeth by instrumentation and the surface polished.

157. Green stain.—The green stain frequently seen on children's teeth may be caused from the decomposition of blood elements or from certain color-producing bacteria. It can readily be removed by applying iodine to the tooth and then polishing with pumice.

Section VI

TECHNIQUE OF DENTAL PROPHYLAXIS

	Paragraph
Instruments	158
Technique	159
System of instrumentation	160
Polishing	161

158. Instruments.—The technique of instrumentation, as described in this manual, will confine itself to instruments available in the Army dental clinics.

a. Mouth mirror.—This instrument is used as—

(1) Reflector of images.
(2) Reflector of light.
(3) Tongue depressor.
(4) Cheek distender.

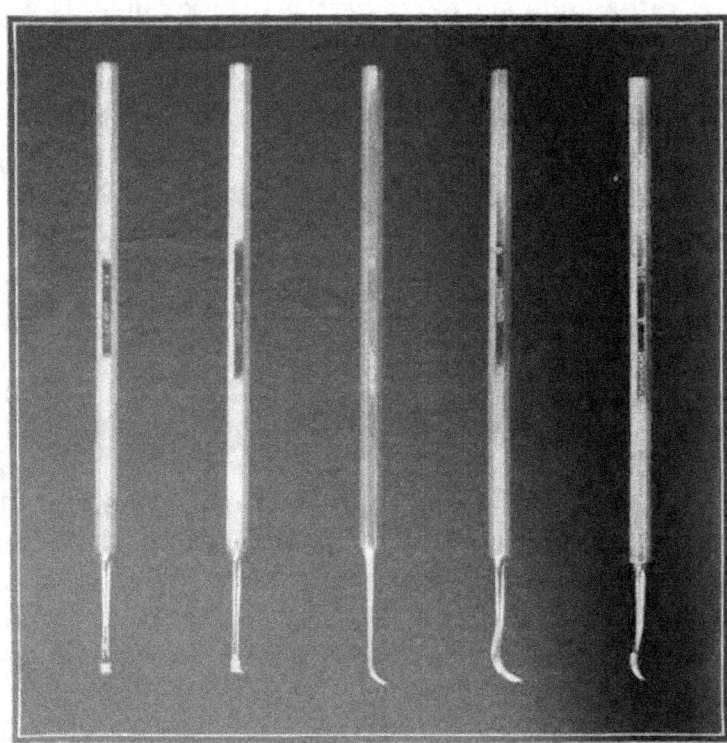

Figure 113.

b. Scalers.—(1) Scalers Nos. 3 and 6 are hooked or sickle-shaped instruments and are used chiefly to remove gross deposits from the teeth. Scaler Younger-Good No. 15 is also sickle-shaped but has a smaller blade and is used to remove small deposits of calculus from more inaccessible places such as between the teeth. Scalers Nos. 33 and 34 are used for the removal of heavy deposits especially from the lingual surfaces of the upper anterior teeth and the lingual surfaces of the lower anterior teeth. The instruments used by the Army dental service (Nos. 3 and 6; Younger-Good Nos. 15, 33, and 34) are all pull instruments (fig. 113), that is, they remove the calculus by a pulling or scraping movement. This type of scaler is called a hoe type for this reason.

(2) Younger-Good No. 15 scaler is used in this operation to check carefully each surface of every tooth to make sure that every piece of calculus has been removed. *It should never be forgotten that all the other pieces of calculus are of minor, even negligible importance as compared with the last piece.*

(3) If the teeth are so shaped or the interproximal span so filled with tissue that the blade does not pass easily around the free margin of the gum *no effort should be used to force the instrument in such a way as to injure the delicate supporting tissues.*

159. Technique.—If the patient presents a mouth in which there is evidence of food debris, the necks of the teeth and the interproximal spaces should be bathed with a solution of hydrogen peroxide. Aside from the germicidal action, the effervescence of the peroxide will mechanically aid in loosening the minute particles of food debris. The mouth should then be rinsed with warm water and then sprayed with a compressed-air atomizer containing a pleasant mouthwash. The air pressure should be at least 25 pounds, so that it will have enough force to blow the spray between the teeth. This premilinary step is very important in mouths of this type as there is danger of infection if instruments are used around the gingival borders where decomposed food is present.

160. System of instrumentation.—In order to perform a prophylactic operation intelligently, one must work by a system and the instrumentation as well as the polishing must have a definite starting point in the mouth and proceed in the same given direction over the surfaces of the teeth in the case of every patient. This is necessary for thoroughness and also useful in case of interruption, for if the operator will make a mental note of the last tooth being worked on when leaving the chair, the chain will remain unbroken on resuming. A good system is to begin on the lingual surface of the right lower last molar and proceed left to the last lower left molar, around to the buccal surface and proceed right to the right lower last molar (fig. 114). The same procedure can be used in the upper jaw. In using instruments in the mouth it must be remembered that each and every motion of the hand and fingers should always be under control of the operator as a slip might cause a great deal of damage to the mouth tissues or the teeth. *An instrument must never be used unless the hand holding it is steadied against some adjoining part of the mouth.* The instrument should be grasped very much the same as a pencil, between the thumb and index finger. The blade of the instrument is placed against the surface of the tooth and is carefully carried under the shoulder of the calculus deposit; with a slight pulling motion of the hand and fingers, and rotating of the wrist, the mass is removed. This same motion is repeated a sufficient number of times to clean thoroughly the surface of the tooth.

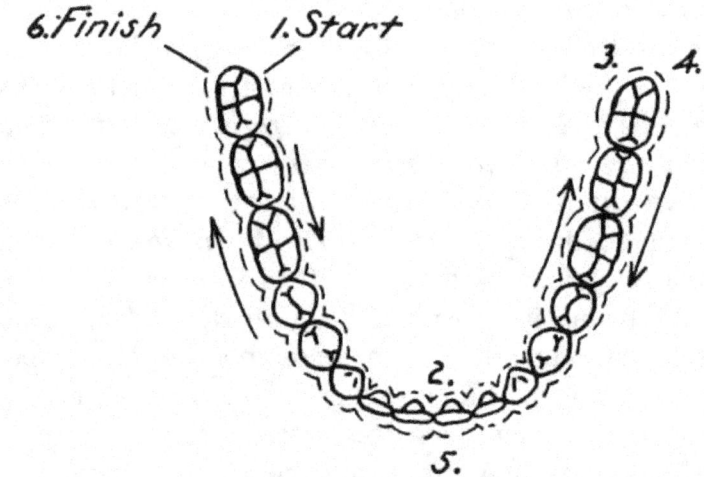

FIGURE 114.—Diagram of dental arch illustrating system of scaling lingual and facial surfaces with definite starting point, procedure, and finishing point which is used on all cases and is conducive to careful yet rapid treatment.

161. Polishing.—*a.* The materials used in polishing the teeth are a contra-angle handpiece and rubber polishing cups. The object of the polishing process is threefold:

(1) Removal of stains, plaques, and films on the exposed surfaces of the teeth.

(2) Polishing of the enamel surfaces and a stimulating effect that seems to be imparted to the living tissues around the tooth by the vigorous massage.

(3) Beneficial results obtained on the gingival margin by the slight pressure from the rubber cup.

b. The main benefit derived from polishing the teeth is the prevention of initial decay.

Section VII

SYSTEM FOR INSTRUMENTATION AND POLISHING

	Paragraph
Instrumentation	162
Polishing	163
Use of dental floss	164
Disclosing solution	165

162. Instrumentation.—The following outline presents a systematic procedure, giving the order in which the different teeth and tooth surfaces are scaled, the scalers used, and the point used to steady the hand holding the instrument (fulcrum point).

a. Division 1.—(1) *Teeth.*—Right lower molars, bicuspids, cuspids, lateral, and central.

(2) *Surface.*—Lingual.

(3) *Instrument.*—Scalers Nos. 3, 6. and 33 (No. 34 also for cuspid, lateral, and central).

(4) *Fulcrum point.*—End of third finger between left lower cuspid and bicuspid on occlusal surface.

b. Division 2.—(1) *Teeth.*—Left lower central, lateral, cuspid, bicuspids, and molars.

(2) *Surface.*—Lingual.

(3) *Instrument.*—Scalers Nos. 3, 6. and 34 (No. 33 also for cuspid, lateral, and central).

(4) *Fulcrum point.*—End of second finger on cutting edge of right lower second bicuspid for left lower central, lateral, and cuspids. End of third finger on cutting edge of lower centrals for bicuspids and molars.

c. Division 3.—(1) *Teeth.*—Left lower molars, biscuspids, and cuspid.

(2) *Surface.*—Buccal.

(3) *Instrument.*—Scalers Nos. 3 and 15.

(4) *Fulcrum point.*—End of third finger on labial surface of lower incisors.

d. Division 4.—(1) *Teeth.*—Lower incisors, right lower cuspid, bicuspids, and molars.

(2) *Surface.*—Facial and buccal.

(3) *Instrument.*—Scalers Nos. 3 and 15.

(4) *Fulcrum point.*—End of second or third finger between left lower cuspid and bicuspid for lower incisors and move posteriorly for molars.

e. Division 5.—(1) *Teeth.*—Right lower molars, bicuspids, and cuspid.

(2) *Surface.*—Approximal.

(3) *Instrument.*—Scaler No. 15.

(4) *Fulcrum point.*—Occlusal surface of right lower bicuspids and move anteriorly for cuspids.

f. Division 6.—(1) *Teeth.*—Lower anteriors.

(2) *Surface.*—Approximal.

(3) *Instrument.*—Scaler No. 15.

(4) *Fulcrum point.*—Occlusal surface of left lower cuspid.

g. Division 7.—(1) *Teeth.*—Left lower cuspids, bicuspids, and molars.

(2) *Surface.*—Approximal.

(3) *Instrument.*—Scaler No. 3 or No. 15.

(4) *Fulcrum point.*—Labial surface of bicuspids and move posteriorly.

h. Division 8.—(1) *Teeth.*—Right upper molars, bicuspids, cuspid, lateral, and central.

(2) *Surface.*—Lingual.

(3) *Instrument.*—Scaler No. 33 (also No. 34 for central, lateral, and cuspid).

(4) *Fulcrum point.*—End of third finger on occlusal surface between left lower cuspid and bicuspid.

i. Division 9.—(1) *Teeth.*—Left upper central, lateral, cuspid, bicuspid, and molars.

(2) *Surface.*—Lingual.

(3) *Instrument.*—Scaler No. 34 (also No. 33 for central, lateral, and cuspid).

(4) *Fulcrum point.*—End of second finger on cutting edge of right upper cuspid.

j. Division 10.—(1) *Teeth.*—Left upper molars, bicuspids, cuspid, lateral, and central.

(2) *Surface.*—Buccal or facial.

(3) *Instrument.*—Scaler No. 3 or No. 34.

(4) *Fulcrum point.*—End of second finger on labial surface of left upper central and lateral and ends of third finger on lingual surface of right upper central and lateral, for molars, cuspids, and bicuspids. End of third finger on cutting edge of right upper cuspid for lateral and central.

k. Division 11.—(1) *Teeth.*—Right upper central, lateral, cuspid, bicuspids, and molars.

(2) *Surface.*—Buccal or facial.

DENTAL TECHNICIANS

(3) *Instrument.*—Scaler No. 3 or No. 33.

(4) *Fulcrum point.*—Back of third or fourth finger on chin.

l. Division 12.—(1) *Teeth.*—Right upper molars, bicuspids, and cuspid.

(2) *Surface.*—Approximal.

(3) *Instrument.*—Scaler No. 3 or No. 15.

(4) *Fulcrum point.*—End of third finger on labial surface of lower incisors.

m. Division 13.—(1) *Teeth.*—Upper incisors.

(2) *Surface.*—Approximal.

(3) *Instrument.*—Scaler No. 15.

(4) *Fulcrum point.*—Incisal edge of upper incisors.

n. Division 14.—(1) *Teeth.*—Left upper cuspid, bicuspids, and molars.

(2) *Surface.*—Approximal.

(3) *Instrument.*—Scaler No. 3 or No. 15.

(4) *Fulcrum point.*—Back of hand resting on chin.

163. Polishing.—The following is a step-by-step outline of the procedure used in polishing the teeth, using a paste of flour of pumice, rubber cups, brush wheels, and the dental engine:

a. Division 1.—(1) *Teeth.*—Right lower molars, bicuspids, and cuspid.

(2) *Surface.*—Lingual.

(3) *Instrument.*—Contra-angle handpiece and rubber cup.

(4) *Fulcrum.*—Lower left second bicuspid.

b. Division 2.—(1) *Teeth.*—Lower anteriors.

(2) *Surface.*—Lingual.

(3) *Instrument.*—Contra-angle handpiece, rubber cup.

(4) *Fulcrum.*—Lower right cuspid.

c. Division 3.—(1) *Teeth.*—Left lower cuspids, bicuspids, and molars.

(2) *Surface.*—Lingual.

(3) *Instrument.*—Contra-angle handpiece, rubber cup.

(4) *Fulcrum.*—Lower right cuspid.

d. Division 4.—(1) *Teeth.*—Left lower molars, bicuspids, and cuspids.

(2) *Surface.*—Buccal.

(3) *Instrument.*—Contra-angle handpiece and rubber cup.

(4) *Fulcrum.*—Incisal edge of lower anteriors.

e. Division 5.—(1) *Teeth.*—Lower anteriors.

(2) *Surface.*—Facial.

(3) *Instrument.*—Contra-angle handpiece and rubber cup.

(4) *Fulcrum.*—Back of hand on chin.

f. Division 6.—(1) *Teeth.*—Right lower cuspid, bicuspids, and molars.

(2) *Surface.*—Buccal.

(3) *Instrument.*—Contra-angle handpiece and rubber cup.

(4) *Fulcrum.*—Back of hand on chin.

g. Division 7.—(1) *Teeth.*—All upper teeth.

(2) *Surface.*—Buccal, facial, and lingual.

(3) *Instrument.*—Contra-angle handpiece and rubber cup.

(4) *Fulcrum.*—Back of hand on chin.

h. Division 8.—(1) *Teeth.*—All molars and bicuspids.

(2) *Surface.*—Occlusal.

(3) *Instrument.*—Straight handpiece and wheel brush.

(4) *Fulcrum.*—Same as for other surfaces of the respective teeth. After the polishing procedure is completed with pumice it can be repeated with powdered chalk to give the teeth a high polish.

164. Use of dental floss.—After the teeth have been polished with cup and brush wheel, there still remain the contact points and areas on the approximal surfaces that have not been reached. These areas are best cleaned with dental floss. A piece of floss about 10 inches long is used for this purpose, and is wrapped around the index finger of one hand and held tightly by the thumb of the other hand. The finger and thumb should not be more than 1 inch apart as this will prevent the floss from snapping against and injuring the gum tissue between the teeth. The dental floss is carefully worked between the teeth and through the contact points until the approximal surfaces of the teeth are reached. It is then drawn over these surfaces several times until all food debris has been loosened and removed. It is then pulled straight out from between the teeth and not past the contact point again. This is repeated between all the teeth, and to facilitate the polishing the floss may be dampened and dipped in pumice before using.

165. Disclosing solution.—*a.* The teeth are then checked for cleanliness by painting a disclosing solution on the dried surfaces. This will make visible all stains and mucinous plaques that have not been removed. A very effective iodine disclosing solution consists of the following:

Iodine crystals	3.3 gm
Potassium iodide	1.0 gm
Zinc iodide	1.0 gm
Glycerin	16.0 cc
Distilled water	16.0 cc

b. A substitute solution of tincture of iodine and glycerin, equal parts, may be used if desired. The patient is allowed to rinse his mouth at frequent intervals during the entire prophylactic treatment. When all the teeth have been thoroughly cleaned and polished, the mouth is sprayed with any pleasant mouthwash.

Section VIII

INSTRUCTIONS TO PATIENT

	Paragraph
Method of tooth brushing	166
Massage	167

166. Method of tooth brushing.—Prevention in dentistry is one of the most important factors to be considered. It is much better to prevent the occurrence of a dental disease than to treat it after it has obtained a start. Probably the most common of all dental conditions is caries or decayed teeth. For a tooth to decay, the process must have a starting point. This is usually brought about by the retention of food debris against the tooth surfaces, which when not removed, will be incorporated into the tartar deposits and, if allowed to remain for several hours, cannot be removed with a brush. Therefore one of the most important duties of the dental hygienist is to understand a good practical method of tooth brushing and to be able to instruct the patient in this method. The instruction will consist of the following: Advise the patient to buy two hard bristle brushes, preferably with different colored handles. One brush to be used in the morning and the other at night. The different colored handles will enable him to know exactly which brush to use. The brushes should be rather small, preferably with two rows of bristles. Place some tooth paste on the dry brush and, using a slight wrist motion, start with the bristles against the gums and sweep them down over the surfaces of the teeth toward the biting edges. The motion should always be from gum to biting surface, and never crosswise. The posterior or back teeth should be brushed first. Then proceed forward until all the teeth are brushed, both inside and out. In this manner, the upper and lower teeth are brushed for 3 minutes by the clock, twice daily. Patients with badly neglected mouths should be told that this manner of brushing might cause their gum tissues to be slightly sore for a day or two, but shortly their mouths will be improved by the massage action of the brush. After the teeth have been thoroughly brushed, there still remain certain areas that are impossible to reach with the brush and must be cleaned with dental floss. Instruct the patient in the use of dental floss as given in paragraph 164.

167. Massage.—Frequently the gums of a neglected mouth will be inflamed and swollen. This condition previously described is known as gingivitis, and can generally be cured or remedied by prophylaxis and massage. Instruct the patient to massage his gums at least twice a day by squeezing or milking the inflamed or soft gums between the ball of the thumb and index finger, downward for the upper arch, and upward for the lower arch. In other words the motion, as in brushing, should always be toward the biting surfaces of the teeth.

Section IX

PREPARATIONS FOR MOUTH AND TEETH

	Paragraph
Oral hygiene	168
Tooth powder and tooth paste	169
Mouthwash	170

168. Oral hygiene.—The science of the health of the mouth treats of the normal equilibrium of the oral cavity and its contents. The medications intended for the maintenance of the health of the mouth and teeth may be divided into those prescribed for specific diseases and those employed as hygienic measures for daily use. Only those employed for hygienic measures are of interest to the dental hygienist.

  a. A good oral preparation should possess the following properties:
  (1) Indifference in regard to—
  (*a*) Mucous membrane (not caustic).
  (*b*) Teeth (nondecalcifying).
  (*c*) Organism as a whole (nonpoisonous).
  (2) Noninterference with the normal physiologic cleansing of the mouth, that is, it must not—
  (*a*) Inhibit the flow of saliva.
  (*b*) Alter or destroy the reaction of the saliva.
  (3) Sufficient cleansing action combined with good taste and odor.
  b. The following should be avoided in constructing a formula for mouth and tooth preparations:
  (1) Strong precipitants of albumen (concentrated alcohol, mineral acids with the exception of boric acid, metallic salts, phenol, and salicylic acid and most of their derivatives, etc.)
  (2) Strong astringents (formaldehyde solution, etc.).
  (3) Caustics (potassium and sodium hydroxide and many of the potassium salts).

(4) Gritty substances (pumice stone, charcoal, crude chalk, etc.).
(5) Fermentable substances (sugars, starches, vegetable powders).
(6) Staining substances (organic and inorganic).

c. Preparations used for the mouth and teeth are conveniently divided into mouthwashes, tooth powders, and tooth pastes.

169. Tooth powder and tooth paste.—Tooth powders and pastes are principally employed for the purpose of mechanically cleansing the accessible surfaces of the teeth. Their antiseptic effect on the bacteria of the mouth is of questionable value, as they remain hardly long enough in the mouth to be completely dissolved. Tooth powders or pastes should not contain gritty or fermentable substances or corrosive chemicals which are destructive to tooth structure. The wasting away of tooth structure, usually referred to as erosion or abrasion, is largely the result of the continuous use of powders, pastes, etc. The principal materials employed in the manufacture of commercial tooth powders and pastes are prepared chalk, precipitated chalk (precipitated calcium carbonate), magnesium carbonate, soap, pumice stone, charcoal, and powdered vegetable drugs such as licorice, orris, myrrh, etc. Prepared chalk and pumice stone are highly abrasive and should never be used in a tooth preparation for daily use. A light preparation of magnesium carbonate has no abrasive or polishing action on tooth structure and is used in the manufacture of tooth powder for bulk. Charcoal is a fine black powder. It should never be used in tooth powder as the sharp particles imbed themselves in the gum tissue producing a bluish line near the free gum margin. A good tooth preparation should contain not more than 2 or 3 percent of the best quality castile soap. Powdered vegetable drugs are added to give flavor and increase bulk, and they can be readily substituted by their respective essential oils. A simple, cheap, effective powder may be made from the following formula: light English precipitated chalk, 94 parts; powdered castile soap, 5 parts; saccharin, $\frac{1}{20}$ part; flavoring, 1 part. A perfectly satisfactory tooth paste cannot be produced without the use of a massing fluid such as gelatin or mucilage of acacia (gum arabic 2 parts, water 3 parts) and glycerin. Tooth pastes may be prepared according to the following formula: tooth powder body, 10 parts; massing fluid, 4 to 6 parts.

170. Mouthwash.—A mouthwash is usually prescribed as a gargle to be used in conjunction with a tooth brush and paste or powder. The components of the wash should be so adjusted that 1 teaspoonful mixed with ½ glass of warm water (approxima 30) furnish the correct proportions of its active ingred most beneficial mouthwash can be made by combining ½ tablespoonful of lime water and ½ teaspoonful of salt to ½ glass of warm water. It acts as a solvent on the mucin deposits on and about the teeth which mechanically retain food debris and bacteria, and its mild astringent effect favors the recovery of inflamed mucous surfaces. This mouthwash corresponds more closely to an artificial saliva, nature's protection of the teeth and mucous membrane, than any mouthwash on the market.

Chapter 6

DENTAL ASSISTANT

	Paragraphs
Section I. Requisites of dental assistant	171–172
II. Care of dental clinic	173–174
III. Sterilization of instruments and dressings	175–181
IV. Care of equipment and supplies	182–190
V. Duties at chair	191–200
VI. Daily routine in clinic	201

Section I

REQUISITES OF DENTAL ASSISTANT

	Paragraph
General	171
Personal hygiene	172

171. General.—*a.* The chair assistant personally associates with all of the patients who receive dental service. The chair assistant directs the patient to the proper chair, sees that the patient is comfortable by adjusting the chair before the dental officer comes into the room, fixes a towel around the patient's neck to protect the clothing, and often arranges appointments for patients. This type of duty demands certain attributes in a dental assistant. First, he must be clean and neat about his person as intimate association with the patients demands this. He must be able to keep the operating room and other rooms of the dental clinic clean and sanitary largely on his own initiative. Finally, he must be respectful, quiet, and dignified, able to arrange appointments courteously with officers, dependents, and enlisted men. In short, the dental assistant must keep himself and the clinic immaculate and must possess the necessary tact to deal with all personnel of the post from the commanding officer down. To carry out these duties successfully, the dental assistant must take pride in his work and must have the greatest respect for the officer for whom he works and for the profession of dentistry. The dental assistant is often the first person whom the patients meet when reporting for dental treatment and their attitude toward the dental service is often influenced by the actions of the dental assistant.

b. Most soldiers presenting themselves for treatment are apprehensive and many are in pain. It is the duty of the dental assistant to see that these patients are assured that they are to receive gentle, scientific treatment, and that their needed dental treatment is nothing to fear. The dental assistant in his duties associates with the varied personnel of the post more often and intimately than any other enlisted member of the Medical Department, and the reputation and good name of the Medical Department enlisted personnel often depend on his manner and attitude.

172. Personal hygiene.—The entire person of the assistant must be scrupulously clean. This means daily baths and change of underwear, a clean regulation uniform at frequent intervals, a daily shave, and frequent haircuts. The hands and nails need particular attention. Before approaching the patient to aid the dental officer always scrub the hands. Let the patient know that this is being done by the thorough use of soap and brush at a basin within his hearing. The nails should be cut close and filed smooth. The orangewood sticks to be found in any office are ideal when properly shaped for cleaning under the nails. After handling infectious material or after handling instruments which were used in treating an infectious disease such as Vincent's infection, special precautions should be used in scrubbing up afterward. One such precaution is to rinse the hands and arms thoroughly in 70 percent alcohol or some similar antiseptic. As to dress, there is no reason why the Medical Department enlisted man should not be as smart in appearance as any enlisted man of the line. The true soldier, with an erect carriage, neat, precise dress, prompt and exact attention to duty, cheerful attitude toward all those who come in contact with him, inspires confidence in the prospective patient. Such a soldier also has confidence in himself.

Section II

CARE OF DENTAL CLINIC

	Paragraph
General	173
Cleaning	174

173. General.—The dental clinic must be kept ready for inspection at all times. There are sufficient cabinets and drawers to keep all instruments and equipment under cover and out of dust and contamination. If tables are used from which to operate, these also may be kept covered with sterile towels or sheets. The assistant should learn where the dental officer habitually keeps his equipment and, after sterilization, should replace it there every time it is used. Many officers like to be able to find things in their offices "in the dark." At least, every officer has a definite place for each item of equipment and it is necessary for the assistant to learn his particular officer's system.

DENTAL TECHNICIANS

174. Cleaning.—*a.* Soap and water and the diligent use of "elbow grease" can keep a clinic spotless at all times. Not only should the floor be scrubbed frequently, but the baseboards, woodwork, cabinets, chairs, waste containers, and similar items of equipment should be scrubbed periodically. The towels or paper covers in the cabinets should be changed at regular intervals or at any time they become soiled. If the floor is waxed, use the proper amount of wax; too much makes it gummy, thus retaining dirt. Such floors should be polished daily. If too much wax has been used and black spots appear, the judicious use of small amounts of kerosene, either alone or to dilute the wax, and hand scrubbing and rubbing will soon remove these spots. Terrazzo floors should never be waxed, but should be scrubbed daily with liberal amounts of soapy water without too much rinsing. The soap thus remaining eventually gives the floor a polished appearance.

b. Windows and glass in cabinets need frequent attention. Door handles and plates or those places most frequently touched in passing through a door must be kept clean, and if metal, must be kept polished.

c. The dental chair must be kept clean and the headrest kept covered with a towel or paper napkin. Paper napkins which are listed on the medical supply table as item No. 73310 are ideal for this purpose when affixed over the headrest cups with rubber bands. When cleaning up, it is a good idea to pump the chair up so that all parts of it can be easily seen and cleaned. As the chair is used so much of the day, special care must be taken to see that it is kept in the best possible condition. It is so constructed that it rarely needs mechanical attention.

d. The unit and especially the cuspidor, must be kept spotless. This last item must be washed after each patient. New covers for the bracket table must be provided for each patient. The water syringe point and the hot air nozzle should be wiped off with 70 percent alcohol after each patient, or these may be disconnected for other means of sterilization, but care must be taken to preserve the gaskets. Any other item on the unit for use in the mouth may be disconnected for sterilization either by chemical means or by boiling.

e. After cleaning everything in the clinic for the day, sit down in the chair and look around; from there, the vantage point of the patient, see what things look like. One will discover things here and there that need going over which were not seen while standing at the chair.

f. Do not overlook the fact that every article of equipment, other than those mentioned, such as tables, desks, waste receptacles, workbench, and washbasin, must be kept clean at all times. The washbasin may have to be cleaned any number of times during the d at the end of the day, it should be thoroughly polished with scouring soap such as Bon Ami; all metal parts should be kept polished at all times. In this connection chrome finished metal needs different care than either nickel or brass. Ask the dental surgeon for instructions on this.

Section III

STERILIZATION OF INSTRUMENTS AND DRESSINGS

	Paragraph
General	175
Bacteriology	176
Sterilizers	177
Sterilizing rules	178
Autoclave	179
Hypodermic syringes and needles	180
Sanitation	181

175. General.—Scientific sterilization of the instruments and dressings used is an essential part of dentistry. Sterilization means the destruction of disease germs and their spores through the agency of heat or chemicals.

176. Bacteriology.—So that the dental assistant will take his responsibility seriously and will be able to work more intelligently, the following brief explanation of disease germs is given:

a. Bacteria are organisms invisible to the naked eye and can be seen only through a microscope. They belong to the plant family and are parasitic, that is, they live on and at the expense of another organism. They cause most of the infections with which dentistry is concerned. Micro-organism, microbe, and **germ are terms** which are sometimes used to mean bacteria.

b. Protozoa are minute organisms somewhat similar to bacteria in that they produce infections and diseases and cannot be seen without the aid of a powerful microscope. However, protozoa belong to the animal kingdom.

c. The two most common classes of bacteria are—

(1) Bacilli (sing., bacillus), rod-shaped organisms when seen under the microscope and some forms produce spores (seedlike forms) which are very hard to kill with heat and chemicals.

(2) Cocci (sing., coccus), round-shaped organisms which, when viewed under the microscope, appear as small dots. This type of bacterium causes most of the infections. It is further classified into a number of subgroups, the chief of which are staphylococcus and streptococcus. The staphylococcus appears under the microscope in clusters and is the cause of most of the pus-forming infections such

as pimples and boils. The streptococcus appears under the microscope in long strings and causes many very serious infections.

177. Sterilizers.—The sterilizers used in the Army are the electric intrument sterilizer and the sterilizing pan containing a strong disinfectant. However, the hospitals will be equipped with a steam-pressure sterilizer called an autoclave. If the dental clinic is large enough it may be equipped with an autoclave and then the dental assistant must familiarize himself with its operation.

178. Sterilizing rules.—The following are some sterilizing rules for instruments, utensils, files, orangewood sticks, etc.:

a. Boil water 15 minutes before starting sterilization.

b. Clean instruments thoroughly with brush, soap, and water (or a 5-percent solution of Lysol) as soon after using as possible. Take special care to brush grooves and joints.

c. Place in sterilizer and boil for 15 minutes.

d. Place all cup-shaped instruments on side or upward so that they will not form air pockets.

e. Never add fresh water to the sterilizer during the sterilizing period and do not add instruments during this period. Either act will contaminate the instrucents already in the sterilizer.

f. At the end of the boiling period, remove the instruments immediately. Sterilized tongs may be used or the instruments may be rolled out on a sterile towel or cloth. Do not touch these instruments with the hands but pick them up with a sterile towel and wipe dry while still warm.

g. These instruments should now be placed in a cabinet with glass trays which are sterilized from time to time.

h. To be completely safe, instruments not recently used should be resterilized before operating (this is especially true in oral surgery).

i. Instruments will not rust if removed and dried immediately after the sterilizing period is up. Allowing them to rest in an elevated tray over boiling water is harmful to them.

j. Never use any form of soda when sterilizing aluminum-handled instruments or when sterilizing hypodermic syringes and needles (a separate sterilizer may be used for these instruments).

k. Although the sterilizer is emptied, scrubbed with soap and water, and dried every evening, a scale from the lime salts in the water will form after a time on the inside of the sterilizer. This should be taken off from time to time by filling the sterilizer with a weak solution of any acid. A little hydrochloric acid well diluted or a cup of vinegar left in the sterilizer overnight will facilitate the removal of this boiler scale.

l. Sharp, fine-edged instruments are damaged by boiling in water. Sterilize these instruments in a compound cresol solution kept in a pan or tray for this purpose. This solution is a liquid containing about 50 percent cresol in a neutral potassium soap and is known by the trade name of Lysol. For the sterilization of instruments, it is used in a dilution of 1 to 3 percent.

179. Autoclave.—The autoclave is an expensive, complicated sterilizing apparatus which sterilizes by the action of live steam. The advantages obtained by the autoclave are: higher temperature can be obtained, and the material sterilized comes from the sterilizer dry and ready to use. Hence this method is used for sterilizing cotton, gauze dressings, gauze and cotton sponges for oral surgery, and cotton points for root canal work. The material to be sterilized, after being prepared according to the directions of the dental officer, is wrapped in muslin and pinned to make a neat and secure pack. These muslin packs are brought to the sterilizing room by the dental assistant for autoclave sterilization. After sterilization, the packs are stored away unopened, and a sterilized reserve of cotton, gauze dressings, gauze and cotton sponges for surgery, and cotton points is always on hand.

180. Hypodermic syringes and needles.—A special sterilizer should be set aside for sterilizing syringes and needles. This sterilizer should not be used for any other purpose and should have careful attention. Syringes and needles should be boiled for 20 minutes. Only distilled water should be used in sterilizing hypodermic needles and syringes. Special care is necessary in the sterilization of needles and syringes because these instruments are used to inject solution deep into the tissues. Any slips in the sterilizing technique of these items will seriously endanger the patient.

181. Sanitation.—Besides actual sterilization of instruments, it is very necessary to maintain ordinary sanitary measures to prevent spread of infection from patient to patient. Most of this sanitary precaution is accomplished in the daily scrubbing and cleaning of the office (see secs. II and IV). However, under the heading of sanitation will come many things too numerous to mention, frequent washing of the operator's and assistant's hands; wearing of clean white gowns or clothing; proper disposal of soiled tongue depressors, cotton rolls, and applicators; use of rubber gloves on luetic patients; and many other simple acts of cleanliness. The dental assistant should develop a sense of asepsis and with some experience should be able to do many things on his own initiative to avoid contamination of equipment and instruments.

DENTAL TECHNICIANS

Section IV

CARE OF EQUIPMENT AND SUPPLIES

	Paragraph
Expendable and nonexpendable property	182
Medicaments	183
Hand instruments	184
Dental burs	185
Engine and handpiece	186
Care of miscellaneous items	187
Dental lathe	188
Vulcanizer	189
Other items	190

182. Expendable and nonexpendable property.—It is most important to know that there are two kinds of equipment in the clinic: expendable and nonexpendable. Expendable equipment consists of those items which are used up in carrying on the work of the clinic such as cement, impression materials, paper cups, paper covers, burs, and similar items. Nonexpendable articles such as hand instruments, forceps, and pliers are charged to the responsible officer and must be accounted for at all times. If nonexpendable equipment breaks or otherwise becomes unserviceable, the parts must be kept and turned in to the hospital medical supply officer for disposal and credit. Nonexpendable property must never be thrown away regardless of its condition. The assistant should ask the officer about each item before it is thrown away until he is thoroughly familiar with these two classes of property. A dental clinic has many, many items of equipment and supply. They are for the most part very expensive and the assistant must learn to take good care of them to prolong their usefulness. Figure 115 shows a supply room with a well-arranged system for storing the different items.

183. Medicaments.—The dental cabinet should contain only those instruments and medicaments that are frequently used. It should never be used as a storage space for surplus supplies as this will only complicate the care of the cabinet. Medicaments are best kept in small, square, ground-glass-stoppered bottles, well labeled with the stock bottle left in the storage room. As the materials are used, they should be replaced from the bulk of the supply. Each bottle should have a certain place in the cabinet and should be kept there when not in use. Number and label the bottles so that the numbers one and two will contain the medicaments most frequently used. They must be spaced on the cabinet shelf so that selected bottles may be removed without tipping one of the others over. In arranging them, it is best not to have medicaments of the same color next to each other. For example eugenol should not be next to phenol. The alcohol bottle may be placed between them. The dan-

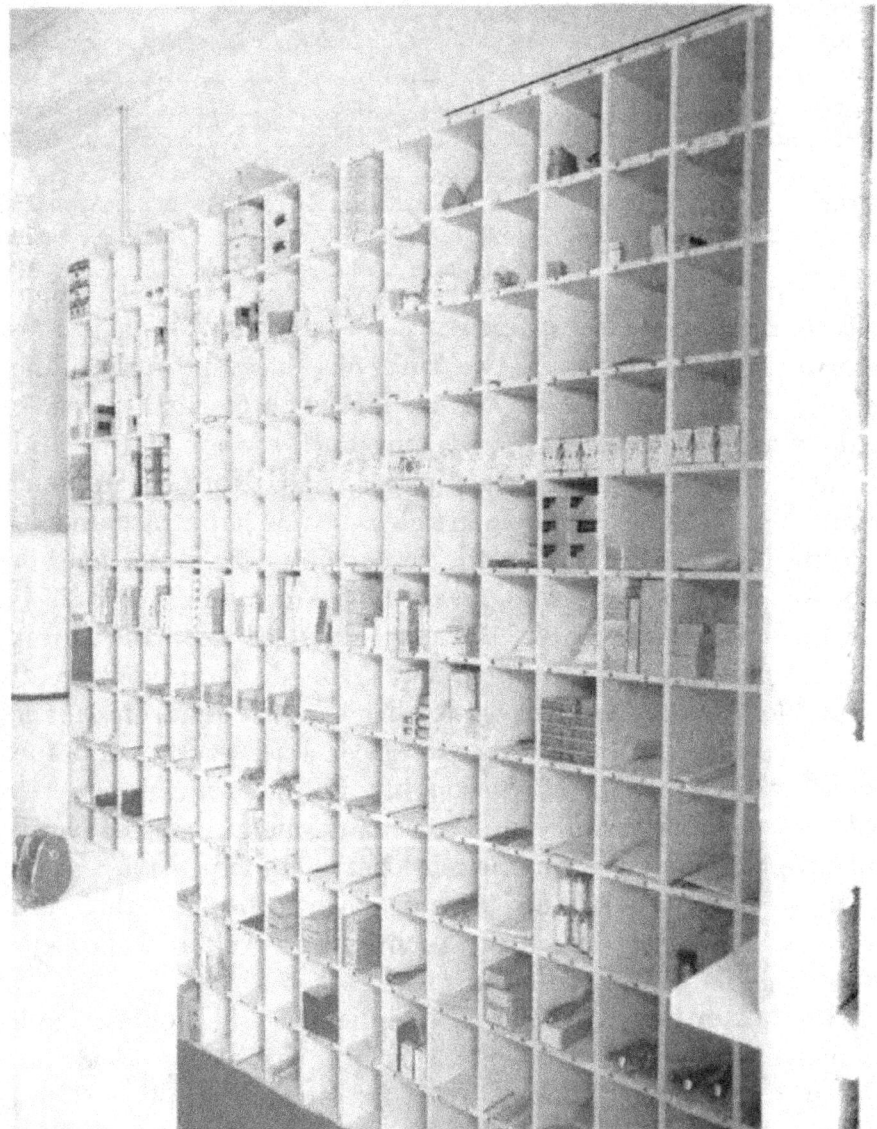

FIGURE 115.—Well-arranged supply room showing how expendable and nonexpendable supplies are stored.

ger of taking the wrong bottle is greatly reduced and the speed in selecting is materially increased. Iodine should not be kept in the cabinet as it will tend to rust the instruments.

184. **Hand instruments.**—Hand instruments should be arranged in the cabinet drawers to suit the dental officer. Each instrument has a definite place. The scalers should be placed together, preferably

pairing the rights and lefts. The same is done with the cutting instruments such as chisels, hatchets, excavators, etc.

185. Dental burs.—The assistant should avoid having a large number of each type and size of burs out in use at one time. With many of the burs partly worn it is difficult for the operator to find a sharp one. Consequently he gets a new one from stock. This is used once and then is placed with the remainder of the old burs and probably never used again. This goes on indefinitely, and consequently many burs that are still serviceable are needlessly thrown away. A very satisfactory method of handling the burs is by the use of any type of bur block that may be available whether it is round or square. The block will contain many holes in which the burs may be placed in regular order. They should be placed so that all types and sizes are readily available but have no more than two or three burs of each kind in the bur block. There are two lengths of burs, those for the straight handpiece and those for the contra-angle handpiece. The burs should be placed so that those for the two handpieces are in the same section of the block for convenience. The different type burs should be placed in groups with the large size burs to the left and graduating down to the small sizes. If after using the bur is still serviceable, it may be cleaned with a wire brush and sterilized and then replaced in the block. If the bur is not serviceable it is thrown away and a new bur replaces it in the bur block. In this manner all the types and sizes of burs are always available and it is a simple matter to replace discarded burs.

186. Engine and handpiece.—The dental engine must be kept clean and free of dust and must be oiled at frequent fixed intervals designated by the dental officer. Oil not only the motor, but the pulleys and the handpieces, using the oil furnished the clinic for this purpose. If the contra-angle is of the all-metal type it should be taken apart and boiled after each period of use and reassembled, using the handpiece grease ("handpiece ease") in all the gears and shafts. *Never use pliers on this handpiece.* With each handpiece furnished, there is a detailed description and cuts showing best how to care for it. Study this and follow the manufacturer's directions. If the handpiece is of the old type that cannot be taken apart and boiled, it should be immersed in a bottle of sterilizing fluid (70 percent alcohol is good) while still on the engine, run forward and backward, then disconnected from the engine and allowed to set in the fluid for a period of sterilization, then removed and oiled; the sheath on the straight handpiece can be boiled, but care must be taken to dry thoroughly the inside of this sheath and in oiling it before replacing it on the handpiece mechanism. It must be remembered that abrasives such as are used for cleaning teeth and polishing restorations are very hard on the handpieces, and great care must be taken to remove thoroughly all particles of pumice or other abrasive when cleaning these handpieces.

187. Care of miscellaneous items.—There are a few items which may be cleaned or cared for in some special way which experience has proved to be best. Impression trays with impression compound adhering to them may be cleaned by applying a liberal coat of vaseline, holding in a flame for a few seconds, and wiping clean with a cloth or paper towel. Plaster bowls and spatulas must be cleaned immediately after use before the plaster or investment material begins to set. This preserves the rubber bowl and makes cleaning these articles easier. Cement slabs and spatulas should also be cleaned immediately after use. This is done by immersing them in a solution of bicarbonate of soda and rubbing the cement off with the fingers before it hardens. By this method the spatula or slab is not scraped and so is kept free from scratches. Extracting forceps will become stiff after being sterilized many times. The joints of these instruments may be loosened by the simple expedient of applying some spirits of ammonia in the joint and working back and forth a few times. The ammonia will loosen any rust in the joint and restore the forceps to their normal usefulness.

188. Dental lathe.—This is another important item in the clinic. It should be kept free from dirt and be cleaned immediately after each period of use. It should be oiled at regular intervals, the frequency depending upon the amount of usage it gets. By carefully cleaning the cup covers before operating them for oiling, no abrasives or foreign materials can get in the bearings. By lightly tapping on the chucks and by removing them by turning the handles mounted on the side of the housing no injury ever will be done to the shafts. With reasonable care this piece of equipment will last many years and is rarely out of order.

189. Vulcanizer.—This is not an item found in many clinics at present, its use being confined to the central dental laboratories. Its care and upkeep are explained in almost any textbook on prosthetic dentistry. Prothero's "Prosthetic Dentistry" has a very good article on the vulcanizer, and the book is found in practically all dental libraries.

190. Other items.—The air compressor is one of the most troublesome items in the clinic. It should be given daily care and inspection. Great care should be taken to see that there are no leaks in the air lines.

It should be shut off or disconnected from the electric current every night. If any unusual knocking is heard or overheating is found, it should be disconnected at once and the dental officer notified. Do not tamper with the pressure-regulating switch unless ordered to do so by the proper authority. Condensation of moisture in the tank causes water to form and this should be drained at regular intervals. This holds true for the lines themselves, there being an outlet at the back of the unit for this purpose. There is a booklet of instructions on the unit in every dental office telling how to take care of it and how to drain the lines as suggested above. If this booklet is misplaced in the office a post card to the company making the unit, stating type, model, and number, will bring this booklet which is invaluable in learning the use and upkeep of all items on the unit. It should be studied thoroughly. All items not in daily use, or those recently obtained from supply sources and not yet opened for use, should be kept in a cool dry place. Instruments or other items liable to rust should be left in their original oilpaper covers or wrapped in oilpaper or gauze covered with petrolatum. If it is possible to have a small storeroom, all items kept in it should be placed on the shelves in numerical order corresponding to the supply table number allotted to that item (fig. 115). This makes for quick inventory and sensible requisition of needed items.

Section V

DUTIES AT CHAIR

	Paragraph
General	191
Handling patients	192
Anesthetic solution	193
Impression materials	194
Filling materials	195
Silver amalgam	196
Copper amalgam	197
Oxyphosphate of zinc cement	198
Silicate	199
Zinc oxide	200

191. General.—During the time that the dental officer is working on the patient the chair assistant should stand by, ready to render any assistance that may be necessary. If there are other duties to be performed in the operating room, he may do them but always within sight of the operator. The best procedure to follow is to stand on the opposite side of the chair from which the operator is working and observe the progress of the work. With a little experience the assistant will be able to anticipate most of the dental officer's wishes and have the necessary instruments ready before they are called for. He should note on the appointment sheet the type of work that is to be done for the patient so that he can have the necessary instruments and materials ready. If it is a prophylaxis, a mouth mirror, scalers, fine pumice, rubber cups, and brush wheels for the handpiece should be placed on the operating tray. If a carious tooth is to be prepared, a mouth mirror, exploring points, handpiece, burs, alcohol, phenol, silver nitrate, etc., should be placed on the tray. This routine is carried out for every patient.

192. Handling patients.—*a.* As brought out in the first section of this chapter the dental assistant comes in closer contact with patients than any other enlisted man in the Medical Department. Many of these patients are suffering actual pain or are in acute discomfort. Do not treat it lightly. This is a serious moment in the patient's day. In all likelihood he approaches the chair in apprehension if not in downright fear. The dental assistant should use the dental surgeon's behavior with patients as a precept of his treatment of them. Remember, there is nothing more painful than an aching tooth, nor anything more uncomfortable than a sore spot under a denture.

b. The main guidepost in handling patients is to conduct oneself as a true gentleman. Be kind and courteous, sympathetic but not gushing, be cheerful and gentle, especially with the timid, be tactful, and show due respect to age and grade. Do not engage in needless and endless conversation with patients. Speak intelligently when spoken to and answer questions when necessary as well as possible although they may seem to be pointless. *Never become familiar.*

c. Telephone calls should be answered in the following manner: "Dental clinic, Private (name) speaking." Get the correct name and the desires of the person calling. If the call is for an appointment, arrange it in consultation with the dental officer; see that it is noted in the appointment book and make sure that the person knows the exact date and hour. If the call is for the dental officer, call him, and if he cannot answer the call, make definite arrangements for completing the call at a later time.

d. Always make definite appointments, exactly recorded on the appointment book and on W. D., M. D. Form No. 65 (Dental Engagement Slip) for patients coming to the clinic for routine appointment. Never give a patient who is suffering pain an appointment for deferred work. Make some arrangement for alleviating the pain.

e. In seating the patient in the chair see that it is in a low comfortable position for the patient, and in a workable position for the dental officer. Be sure the headrest is comfortable and has a clean cover; place a clean towel on the patient, and secure it about the neck with the holder. Then wash the hands before placing a clean mirror, explorer, and cotton pliers on the bracket table. The patient's W. D., M. D. Form No. 79 (Register of Dental Patients) is placed on the desk, and the patient is ready for the dental officer.

193. Anesthetic solution.—*a.* Ringer's solution may be made up in 100-cc lots as often as necessary. Equipment necessary for making the anesthetic solution is dissolving cup with holder, procaine tablets, sterile gauze, alcohol or gas flame, and a 10-cc graduate with straight sides. As this solution is to be injected into the patient it is absolutely necessary for it to be sterile. Any carelessness on the part of the assistant might endanger the life of the patient. The dental officer will state how many cubic centimeters of anesthetic solution he wants. If 3 cc are desired, three tablets of procaine hydrochloride are emptied from the little vial upon the sterile gauze. They should not be touched by the hands at any time. The use of cotton pliers is indicated in the handling of the tablets. Measure 3 cc of Ringer's solution in the graduate and pour into a clean dissolving dish. Heat the solution over the flame until it reaches the boiling point. Drop into the solution the three tablets of procaine and heat a little more until they are completely dissolved. The solution is now ready to be placed in the syringe. Since it is convenient not to remove the needles from the syringe once they are placed on, two syringes should be available, one having the $1\frac{5}{8}$-inch needle, and the other syringe equipped with the 1-inch needle. Take whichever syringe is indicated from the cabinet, and remove the little piece of wire that is placed through the needle. This is carefully laid to one side where it can be found again after the syringe has been used. Place the needle in the solution and draw up until the syringe is filled with anesthetic solution. Place the barrel of the syringe against the inside of wrist to test for temperature. The ideal temperature for the solution is about body temperature. The needle is then passed several times through the flame until it becomes slightly red in color. This can only be done with iridio-platinum needles, however, and if steel needles are used they should not be flamed. Hold the syringe so that the needle is pointing upward and slowly push the plunger until all the air has been expelled from the syringe. It is then handed to the dental officer or placed on the operating tray, taking precautions so that the needle does not touch anything. If this happens it is necessary to reflame the needle before using. After the syringe has been used, the plunger is removed from the barrel, the wire is placed in the needle, and the entire syringe is placed in the sterilizer and boiled for a minimum of 15 minutes. After sterilizing, the syringe is assembled and placed back in the cabinet where it is ready to be used again.

b. Cartridge-type syringes are now available, and if this type of local anesthetic equipment is in use in the clinic, the sterilization and preparation are much simplified. The anesthetic solution comes in a sealed glass cartridge which is placed in a sterile syringe with the needle affixed. The cartridge containing the sterile solution becomes the barrel of the syringe. In using this type of syringe, the needle and syringe must be sterilized immediately before the injection. The needles should be sterilized in a separate compartment and should not be touched by hand after sterilizing. These needles are rustless steel and should *never be flamed*.

c. The syringe should be completely disassembled periodically, scrubbed, cleaned thoroughly, and a drop of light oil applied to the plunger bearing to assure its mechanical efficiency.

194. Impression materials.—If an impression is to be taken, the necessary impression materials will be made available, depending upon the type of impression. If modeling compound is used, the assistant should place a pan of water over the fire and heat it until the water is just a little too warm to allow the hand to be kept in the water. Several cakes of modeling compound are laid on a clean towel beside the hot water. The tray that has been selected by the dental officer is oiled slightly over its outer surface. If a hydrocolloid material is used, it is necessary to heat the pan of water to the boiling point. After the tray has been selected and attached to the water connections of the unit by rubber tubing, the stick of hydrocolloid material is placed in the boiling water. The manufacturer's directions are followed as to the length of time that it is to be heated, but it is usually about 8 minutes. The tube containing the softened material is removed from the hot water and placed in water that is lukewarm. The tube is kneaded between the fingers for a minute and then placed against the wrist to test the temperature. When it is warm but not uncomfortable it is ready to be taken into the operating room for use by the dental officer.

195. Filling materials.—The mixing of the various dental filling materials is one of the most important duties of the chair assistant. The durability and appearance of the filling will depend upon its proper manipulation during this stage. Several types of materials are used: gold, silver amalgam, oxyphosphate, copper amalgam, zinc oxide, silicate, gutta percha, etc. The filling materials that the chair assistant must prepare are known as plastics; that is, they are prepared and inserted while in a plastic stage and become hard after being placed in the tooth. This includes the amalgams and silicates which are known as permanent filling materials, and also oxyphosphate, zinc oxide, and gutta percha which are known as the temporary filling materials.

196. Silver amalgam.—The most common type of material used is the silver amalgam. It consists of the powdered metal portion containing silver, tin, and copper. This is mixed with mercury in the proportion of seven parts of alloy to five parts of mercury by weight or according to the manufacturer's directions. The mixture is placed in a glass mortar and triturated for 3 minutes or until the particles of metal have been thoroughly incorporated into the mercury. The mix is then placed in the palm of one hand and using the thumb of the other hand, it is thoroughly mixed until the material gives a slight metallic sound. Excess mercury should be expressed from the amalgam by the operator.

197. Copper amalgam.—Copper amalgam comes in small pellets with the mercury already included in the material. The pellet is placed in a spoon and heated slightly over a flame until the amalgam becomes soft. It is then placed in a mortar and triturated as was the silver amalgam. The excess amalgam left after the filling is inserted may be saved and used again.

198. Oxyphosphate of zinc cement.—Oxyphosphate of zinc cement can be used as a temporary filling material or as a cement for gold crowns and inlays. The consistency of the mix should vary slightly according to the use to which it is put. If it is to be used for cementing crowns and inlays, the cement should be of a rather thin consistency so that it will occupy a minimum of space under the filling. If it is to be used as a filling material it should be mixed a little heavier in order to obtain a greater degree of strength for the filling. The more powder used in the mix, the stronger the cement will be. The powder comes in various shades ranging from dark yellow to snow white. When the shade of the powder is determined by the dental officer three small portions of the powder are placed on a clean glass slab. Three or more drops of the phosphoric acid liquid are placed on the slab about 1 inch away from the powder. Using a small metal spatula, the powder is gradually incorporated into the liquid, adding small portions of powder at a time and spatulating thoroughly. If the powder is added too fast, the mix will become hard and unmanageable as the setting time will be decreased. Continue adding small portions of powder and spatulating with a rotary motion until the cement has a tendency to string out from the spatula when it is raised and then falling back, forming a little mound which retains its shape. A great deal of practice will be required before the proper mixture can always be obtained. The chair assistant should always mix the cement under the supervision of the dental officer until he has attained this proficiency.

199. Silicate.—The silicates or synthetic porcelain filling materials require the greatest care in mixing. There are so many variable factors which influence the silicates that the most rigid routine must be followed. The silicate powders come in numerous shades, each one having a number. The desired shade is determined by the dental officer from the silicate shade guide. The shade decided upon, the next step is to make certain that all the equipment necessary for the filling is ready. None of the materials such as glass slabs, spatulas, etc., should be used for any other purpose than for silicate fillings. The metal spatula for mixing and the plastic instruments used in inserting the filling in the tooth are made from a special alloy, either stainless steel or stellite. As the various powders may be mixed to give the exact shade desired, a special silicate shade guide is used on which are given the correct proportions of each powder to obtain this shade. Some of the shades will require an even mix of two powders and other shades will require one portion of one powder to two portions of another shade. Each silicate set contains a metal scoop used to determine the correct amount of the powder. This scoop has small spoonlike ends, one end smaller than the other. The small end is used to measure the powder when a mix calls for one portion of one powder to two portions of another powder. The larger end is used to measure the powder when the mix calls for equal portions of two powders. Depending upon the shade selected, the powder is measured as directed, and placed upon a clean, dry glass slab. A word of warning about the slab: In hot weather the slab should first be cooled with cold water and dried before attempting to mix the silicate. The ideal temperature is between 65° and 75° F. Moisture of any sort will affect the strength of the final filling. The silicate set contains a box of celluloid strips. One or two of these strips are placed upon the operating tray. They will be used by the dental officer as a matrix in the insertion of the filling. Three full drops of the liquid are always used when the powder is measured out as directed. These three drops are placed on the glass slab about an inch away from the powder. Add about one-third of the powder to the liquid and spatulate for not more than 20 seconds. Add another third of the powder and spatulate for the same time. The final third of the powder is then added and the spatulation is completed when the mixture has the consistency of soft putty. The entire mix should never be spatulated for more than 1 minute, and the spatulation should be done lightly, using a patting motion instead of the rotary motion used in mixing cements.

200. Zinc oxide.—Zinc oxide and eugenol are used extensively as a temporary filling material because of their sedative action. Three or more drops of eugenol are placed on a glass slab. Enough zinc oxide powder is placed on the slab for that particular filling. The powder is incorporated into the eugenol with a metal spatula until it is thoroughly mixed. The resultant mixture is rolled into a small ball and squeezed between two pieces of gauze, thus expressing some of the oil. When the mixture is of the proper consistency for insertion in the cavity, it is placed on the operating tray.

Section VI

DAILY ROUTINE IN CLINIC

	Paragraph
General	201

201. General.—*a.* If some routine schedule can be followed each morning before the actual work in the clinic begins, nothing will be overlooked and this daily, rather monotonous task will be made to pass quickly. Therefore the following schedule is suggested: In the morning, thoroughly air the clinic; turn on appliances on units; start water running in the cuspidors; fill and start the sterilizer; start the air compressor; attend to the linen supply; fold towels and place them in cabinets; check spray bottles; have soap and towels at all wash basins; check paper towel and paper cup supply; assemble W. D., M. D. Form No. 79's for the day's appointments; if the type of work to be done is known, make the initial preparations for the first patient; have a clean gown in readiness for the dental officer; make a final check for dust. During the noon hour, sweep out the clinic; rearrange office, desk, and waiting room. At the end of the day, thoroughly clean and dust the clinic; rearrange office and waiting room; drain and clean the sterilizer; turn off all water, gas, and electricity; check and record all Form No. 79's; record all changes in classification; file the day's records and X-rays; empty all wastecans; get linen ready for exchange in the morning; and check all medicine bottles, refilling if necessary.

b. In addition to the routines mentioned, it is usually the duty of the dental assistant to close the office each evening. Elevate the chairs close and lock all windows, see that all water has been turned off, see that all electric switches have been turned off (*it is especially important to make sure that the sterilizers are turned off*), see that the safe is locked, and on the way out see that all doors are locked.

Chapter 7

RECORD CLERK, DENTAL SERVICE

	Paragraphs
Section I. General duties and forms used	202–205
II. W. D., M. D. Form No. 57 (Report of Dental Service)	206–207
III. W. D., M. D. Form No. 79 (Register of Dental Patients)	208–210
IV. W. D., M. D. Form No. 18b (Statement of Expenditure of Special Dental Materials)	211–213
V. Daily work sheet	214
VI. Hospital clinic records	215–219
VII. W. D., A. G. O. forms	220–221
VIII. Dental survey	222–224
IX. Dental history of station	225–227

Section I

GENERAL DUTIES AND FORMS USED

	Paragraph
Routine reports	202
Other forms used	203
Record of annual dental survey	204
Appointment book	205

202. Routine reports.—There are three principal reports and records that are routinely required from all stations where a complete dental service is maintained. These are as follows:

a. W. D., M. D. Form No. 57 (Report of Dental Service).—This is a report required monthly from every station where a dental surgeon is on duty and from every tactical unit having a dental officer assigned. This report is signed by the dental surgeon, indorsed by the surgeon, and forwarded to higher authority in compliance with existing directives. It is explained in detail in section II.

b. W. D., M. D. Form No. 79 (Register of Dental Patients).—This is the patient's card, and one is made for each individual admitted to the dental clinic. These reports are filed permanently in the hospital and under present regulations are not forwarded. It is taken up in detail in section III.

c. W. D., M. D. Form No. 18b (Statement of Expenditure of Special Dental Materials).—This form, together with Form No. 57, is forwarded monthly from all stations or commands having dental laboratory facilities. Where dental work is accomplished with only chest No. 60, M. D., as in the dispensaries of tactical units, this form need not be forwarded. It is explained in detail in section IV.

203. **Other forms used.**—*a.* W. D., M. D. Form No. 65 (Dental Engagement Slip) is the appointment card. It should be given the patient for every appointment made for him at the clinic. The patient should be instructed to give the card to his first sergeant immediately so that he will be excused at the proper time for the appointment. A better way to arrange for appointments is to send this form through post headquarters to the individual's organization. In this way it becomes an order for the individual to report at the dental clinic at the specified time.

b. W. D., M. D. Forms Nos. 16a, 16b, 16c, and 16d are property forms and are all similar except that they are used for different purposes. Form No. 16a is a request for expendable medical property; Form No. 16b is a request for issue of nonexpendable medical property; Form No. 16c is a credit slip for nonexpendable property turned in to the medical supply officer; and Form No. 16d is a request for exchange of nonexpendable medical property. These four forms are used when requisitioning property, turning in property, or exchanging property. They are initiated in the dental clinic and forwarded to the hospital medical supply officer for action.

c. W. D., M. D. Form No. 124 (Prosthetic Case Record) is filled out in duplicate and mailed with each case sent to the central dental laboratory. W. D., M. D. Forms No. 123 (Label, Penalty) is merely an address sticker to apply to mailing cases when sending them to the central dental laboratory. These last two forms are obtained from the central dental laboratory.

d. All other forms are obtained by the medical supply officer from the medical supply depot on semiannual requisition.

204. **Record of annual dental survey.**—This is a record of vital importance in the clinic. It is a complete roster of all military personnel of the command with their grade, age, organization, nativity, length of service, and dental classification. The Army classification of I, II, III, IV is used, indicating relative urgency for dental treatment. The dental officer will explain exactly what is meant by these four classifications.

205. **Appointment book.**—The appointment book is the dental officer's work schedule. Record every appointment made; write plainly the grade, name, and hour. Always consult the dental officer about appointments, if possible, before making them.

DENTAL TECHNICIANS

TM 8-225
206

Section II

W. D., M. D. FORM NO. 57 (REPORT OF DENTAL SERVICE)

	Paragraph
General	206
Daily compilation of Form No. 57	207

206. General.—Although Form No. 57 is rendered monthly, all the admissions, sittings, changes in classification, and work accomplished must be recorded on the form daily so that at the end of the month the form will be up to date and will only need to be typed in good form to be completed. The method of daily recording the work on Form No. 57 from the patient's cards is explained later in this section. The completed form will conform to the following:

a. Paragraph 1.—State station or command to which assigned or attached for duty with its location. If the dental service is with a tactical unit, state the number and name of the division, regiment, or other unit with its location as the case may be.

b. Paragraph 2.—Give the month or the beginning and end of period if less than the calendar month. This should only cover a single calendar month. If the period is less than a month but extending into a second calendar month, say from June 20 to July 3, two reports must be made out and forwarded. one from June 20 to June 30 and another from July 1 to July 3. However, most dental clinics will be functioning indefinitely and reports will be made out for the whole calendar month each month.

c. Paragraph 3.—The same as paragraph 1, plus any additional stations or commands which were provided regular and routine treatment. Others receiving treatment, Civilian Conservation Corps patients or any other nonmilitary personnel should *not* be listed under this paragraph.

d. Paragraph 4.—(1) *Admissions, routine, military.*—Record total admissions of military personnel admitted for treatment as a routine procedure.

(2) *Admissions, emergency, military.*—Record total admissions of military personnel admitted for the relief of pain or other intolerable conditions. A case may be admitted but once. If a case is not completed during one calendar month, it is not recorded as an admission for the following month. If a case is discontinued, interrupted, or postponed for an indefinite period and the patient later returns for further treatment, it may be recorded as a new admission at the discretion of the dental officer concerned who will be governed by the elapsed time and circumstances of the case.

(3) *Sittings given, military.*—Each visit of a patient to a dental office for treatment is considered a sitting. Sittings for purpose of examination should be recorded.

(4) *Others.*—All three headings are to be divided into two parts. The admissions and sittings for Civilian Conservation Corps enrollees are entered in right-hand column so formed, and those for all "others" are entered in left-hand column so formed.

e. Paragraph 5.—(1) *Initial classification.*—When an annual survey or any other complete survey of the command covered by the report is made, the results of the survey are entered as the initial classification. Otherwise, the final classification of the previous monthly report is entered as the initial classification of the current report. When an initial classification resulting from a complete survey is entered, all previous tabulations in paragraph 5 will be dropped and a new tabulation will be initiated.

(2) *Additional classification.*—Enter the results of any partial surveys covering personnel not present for previous surveys. Enter classification of personnel applying for treatment who have not been classified by survey.

(3) *Changes in classification.*—(a) When a patient's classification is changed as the result of work accomplished, enter in appropriate plus and minus columns. Example: A class I case which has been completed to class IV will be entered as "1" on the minus line under class I and also as "1" on the plus line under class IV.

(b) The total of the initial classifications, the additional classifications, and the plus classifications should be entered on the line provided between the plus and minus lines.

(4) *Final classification.*—(a) Subtract the figures in the minus columns from the totals of the initial, additional, and plus classifications and enter these as the final classifications.

(b) It is recognized that changes in personnel are frequent and that the classification will not be entirely accurate. However, certain valuable statistical data can be obtained from the figures given which will be relatively accurate. To obtain greater accuracy, the dental service under favorable conditions may be able to check the transfers of personnel from the station and drop those transferred from their surveys. Under the same circumstances all new arrivals could also be checked, surveyed, and listed under additional classifications. Wherever this procedure is established, those transferred permanently from the command should be dropped by entry below the final classification. Subtraction of these figures from the final classification fig-

DENTAL TECHNICIANS

ures will then provide a corrected final classification which in turn becomes the initial classification of the following month (fig. 116).

5. CLASSIFICATION OF MILITARY PERSONNEL

	Class I	Class II	Class III	Class IV
Initial classification	300	600	50	400
Additional classification	40	50	5	55
Changes in classification — Plus		30	2	50
Changes in classification	340	680	57	505
Changes in classification — Minus	42	37	3	
Final classification	298	643	54	505
Transferred from command	10	20		15
Corrected final classification	288	623	54	490

FIGURE 116.

f. Paragraphs 6 and 7.—(1) These two parts of the form are recorded from paragraphs 10 and 11 of Form No. 79, the patient's card, a form which is completed for each patient recording the disease or injury and the operation performed. The manner in which this is accomplished is explained later in this section.

(2) Most of the diagnoses and operations performed are self-explanatory as listed on the Form No. 57, but a few may be misinterpreted. Enter after "mandible edentulous" and "maxillae edentulous" only those cases for which replacements have been inserted during the current month. Thus, if 7 partial dentures replacing a total of 40 missing teeth and 6 bridges replacing a total of 12 missing teeth were inserted during the month reported, the total after tooth missing should be 52. Do not enter teeth replaced by full dentures under tooth missing.

(3) The dental clinic in which the impression is taken and the appliance inserted will take credit for such denture, bridge, or repair.

(4) Divide the "others total" column into two parts in both paragraph 6 and 7 and enter CCC at the head of the right-hand column so formed. Record totals for Civilian Conservation Corps enrollees in this column and the totals for all "others" in left-hand column so formed.

TM 8-225
206   MEDICAL DEPARTMENT

(5) In paragraph 7 restorations of a temporary nature should not be entered but should be considered as treatments. Thus, there should be no entry after "gutta percha" nor should "zinc oxide and eugenol" be entered as an addition to the column of restorations.

(6) In the blank spaces under the last printed entry in paragraph 7, a list of causes of extractions should be made.

DUTY PERSONNEL

8. COMMISSIONED

Mean strength   Assigned_____

Number of dental officers on duty_____ Attached_____ Total days of duty_____

9. ENLISTED

Name	Grade	Special Qualifications	Rating	Efficiency

FIGURE 117.

g. Paragraph 8.—(1) *Number of dental officers on duty.*—(a) Due to the probable fluctuation of officers on duty both assigned and attached, particularly in the large clinics, only a figure showing the mean strength of each will be of value. Consequently, over "number of dental officers on duty" type the words "mean strength." Then type two headings, "assigned" and "attached" (fig. 117).

(b) To compute the mean strength for each group, add the number of days each officer was assigned or attached to the organization during the month. Example: To compute mean strength of assigned officers in a clinic to which ten officers have been assigned during the month—five on duty the full month, two for 15 days, two for 10 days, and one for 5 days.

Computation:

$$5 \times 30 = 150$$
$$2 \times 15 = 30$$
$$2 \times 10 = 20$$
$$1 \times 5 = 5$$

Total days $205 \div 30 = 6.8$ mean strength

(c) Repeat the same procedure to obtain mean strength of attached officers.

(2) *Total days of duty.*—Take the total days figures from the computations used in determining mean strengths of assigned and attached officers and deduct days lost from duty. Example: In (1) above the total days figure for assigned personnel is 205. Assume that the figure for attached personnel was 150. Then the total assigned or attached days was 355. One officer was sick in hospital 10 days and one for 12 days. One officer was on leave of absence for 8 days. Thus, 30 days were lost from duty. 355 minus 30 equals 325 days of duty.

h. Paragraph 9.—(1) Enter permanently assigned enlisted personnel only, as of last day of month.

(2) Following last entry of assigned enlisted personnel type in: "Enlisted personnel attached from other units, mean strength."

(3) Next list all civilian personnel by occupation, that is, hygienists, chair assistants, dental mechanics, etc.

(4) If space is insufficient, paste an additional sheet at bottom of page. When completed, fold upward over face of form carrying paragraphs 8 and 9.

i. Paragraph 10.—(1) List all dental officers assigned to unit or units covered by the report giving grade, name, status (RA, Res, NG), duty performed, dates of leave, detached service, sick in hospital, etc.

(2) Following last entry of assigned officer personnel, type in "Officer personnel attached from other units.

(3) Record the amount of time devoted to purely instructional purposes by both officers and men. Example:

	Hours
Instruction of officers	12
Instruction of enlisted men	9

(4) Record all conditions which interfere with or diminish the amount of professional service during the month such as lack of suitable equipment or supplies, lack of availability of military personnel for treatment, or other adverse conditions.

(5) For additional space, paste an additional sheet above the word "certificate" so that paragraph 11 and its contents are not permanently covered.

207. Daily compilation of Form No. 57.—As was brought out in paragraph 206, the information on Form No. 57 must be kept from day to day, although the completed report is forwarded only once a

TM 8-225
207　　　　　　　　MEDICAL DEPARTMENT

month. It was also stated that the information for Form No. 57 was obtained from Form No. 79. The simplest and easiest way for the record clerk to obtain and record this information is as follows:

a. Each officer will keep a daily work sheet on which the officer records all of the diseases or injuries treated and the operations performed for each patient.

b. At the end of the day the record clerk collects these daily work sheets from each officer and records the operations performed for that day upon each individual patient's Form No. 79.

c. On a Form No. 57, used for this purpose, each card (Form No. 79) is taken in turn, and the information from the card is recorded on the Form No. 57.

d. The information transferred in this way completes paragraph 4. the changes in classification part of paragraph 5, paragraph 6, and paragraph 7. Each patient who has a card made out for him on that day is entered as a sitting. Each change in classification appearing on the cards is entered once as minus in the old classification and once as plus in the new classification. Paragraphs 10 and 11 on Form No. 79 correspond, respectively, with paragraphs 6 and 7 on Form No. 57. All the notations under paragraphs 10 and 11 are transferred to paragraphs 6 and 7 on Form No. 57. The best way to record these admissions, changes in classification, cases diagnosed, and operations performed is by using small tally marks on the Form No. 57 for each entry on the patient's card. At the end of the month these tally marks are added, and the total obtained is entered on the Form No. 57 which is to be forwarded. Figure 118 shows a Form No. 79 properly filled out and figure 119 shows paragraphs 6 and 7 of Form No. 57 with these data transferred.

DENTAL TECHNICIANS

REGISTER OF DENTAL PATIENTS AT
FORT BLANK, VIRGINIA

(1) Surname	(2) Christian name
Jones, Charles G.–15792486	

(3) Rank	(4) Company	(5) Regiment or Staff Corps
Pvt.	B	4th Engrs.

(6) Age years	(7) Race	(8) Nativity	(9) Service, years
24	W	Virginia	2–4/12

(10) Disease or injury with location, complications, sequelae, etc.	(11) Dates and nature of treatments and operations	(12) Results and remarks
Abscess parietal, acute, R14	1941	
	Feb. 3–AInc	Emergency, Ad Cl I
Crs R13 mo	Feb. 4–GT	Cl I to II
Crs L13 do	Feb. 20–A	
Crs L14 o	Feb. 24–A	
Crs L15 mo	Feb. 28–A	
Crs L9 m	Feb. 28–OA	Cl II to III
Maxilla edentulous	March 3–S	
	March 18–Denture Upper, Vulcanite	Cl III to IV

Charles F. Smith
Charles F. Smith, Major

Dental Corps, U. S. A.

Form 79—Medical Department, U. S. A.
(Revised Feb. 24, 1941)

Figure 118.

CASES DIAGNOSED AND OPERATIONS PERFORMED

6. CASES DIAGNOSED					7. OPERATIONS PERFORMED		
	PATIENTS					PATIENTS	
	Military		Others				
Diagnoses	Primary disease	Total	Primary disease	Total	Nature of operations	Military, total	Others, total
1. Abscess, parietal		1			RESTORATIONS		
2. Abscess, periapical							
3. Abrasion					Amalgam	3	
4. Adenitis					Gold, foil		
5. Ankylosis, bony					Gutta-percha		
6. Ankylosis, fibrous					Inlay		
7. Bridge, defective					Inlay recemented		
8. Calculus					Oxyphosphate		
9. Caries		5			Oxyphosphate and amalgam	1	
10. Cellulitis					Root canal		
11. Cleft-palate					Silicate	1	
12. Crown, defective							
13. Cyst, dentigerous							
14. Cyst, radicular							
15. Denture, defective							
16. Erosion							
17. Filling, defective					PROSTHESES		
18. Fracture of mandible					Bridge (all types)		
19. Fracture of maxilla					Bridge, recemented		
20. Fracture of tooth					Bridge, repaired		
21. Gingivitis					Crown (all types)		
22. Hypercementosis					Crown, recemented		
23. Leukoplakia					Crown, repaired		
24. Malocclusion					Denture (all types)	1	
25. Mandible, edentulous					Denture, adjusted		
26. Mandible, necrosis of					Denture, rebased		
27. Maxillae, edentulous		1			Denture, repaired		
28. Maxilla, necrosis of					Splint		
29. Neuralgia, facial							
30. Osteitis							
31. Osteomyelitis							
32. Periodontitis							
33. Periodontoclasia					OTHER OPERATIONS		
34. Periostitis					Abscess, incision of	1	
35. Pulp, devitalization of					Alveolectomy		
					Anesthesia, general		
36. Pulpitis							
37. Sequestrum					Anesthesia, local		
38. Sinusitis					Apicoectomy		

FIGURE 119.

6. CASES DIAGNOSED					7. OPERATIONS PERFORMED		
	PATIENTS					PATIENTS	
	Military		Others				
Diagnoses	Primary disease	Total	Primary disease	Total	Nature of operations	Military, total	Others, total
39. Stomatitis, apthous					Calculus, removal of		
40. Stomatitis, catarrhal					Examination		
41. Stomatitis, mercurial					Fracture, reduction of		
42. Stomatitis, ulcerative					Gingiva-alveolus, debridement of		
43. Stomatitis, syphilitic					Gums, excision of		
					Gums, treatment of	1	

FIGURE 119—Continued.

SECTION III

W. D., M. D., FORM NO. 79 (REGISTER OF DENTAL PATIENTS)

	Paragraph
Personal data	208
Recording diseases and treatments	209
Filing	210

208. Personal data.—Form No. 79 is the individual patient's record which remains on file in the dental clinic. When a patient reports at the clinic for the first time, a Form No. 79 is prepared for him before any dental operations are started. Uniformity in the preparation of the form is very important. The patient's last name, first name, middle initial, and Army serial number should be entered on the first line of the register in that order. On the second line the grade, company, and regiment or arm or service are entered for enlisted personnel; the grade and arm or service will be entered for commissioned officer personnel. For all cards on others receiving treatment, this line will be used to record their connection with the Military Establishment, such as civilian employee, Quartermaster Corps; civilian, wife of major, Infantry; or civilian, WPA worker. On the third line, paragraph 6, the age at the nearest birthday is required. In paragraph 8 the State or country, if other than the United States, in which the patient was born is entered. In paragraph 9, the years' service is entered as years and monthly fractions of a year such as $2^{6}/_{12}$, $3^{4}/_{12}$, etc.

209. Recording diseases and treatments.—Paragraphs 10, 11, and 12 of this card are used to record the diseases treated and the operations performed. The standard terms for diagnosis and the abbreviations which are permitted are given in AR 40-1010. The date treatment is given is entered under paragraph 11. The year may be entered at the head of the column at the left side just above the first line (fig. 118). Under paragraph 12 type of admission is entered, either routine or emergency, and the classification. Any subsequent changes in classification are also entered in this section.

210. Filing.—When a patient is confined to quarters or hospital as a result of dental conditions, the dental surgeon will furnish the surgeon with a duplicate of the patient's case record, Form No. 55E-5. When a patient is referred to a dental clinic by a medical officer for treatment, a duplicate of the patient's case record, showing treatments given and operations performed, will be furnished the commanding officer of the hospital for incorporation in the patient's clinical record. When space provided on the card is insufficient to complete the record of a case, an additional card will be fastened to it and entries continued thereon. The register cards will be kept in two files, the current file and the permanent file. The current file will consist of register cards of patients whose case records are not closed; the cards will be arranged alphabetically, according to the surnames of the patients. The permanent file will comprise all register cards of closed cases. The cards will be arranged alphabetically in the same manner as cards in the current file. The permanent file will be kept yearly, a new file being started January 1 of each year. The cards of the old year's file will then be placed with the dental history of the station.

Section IV

W. D., M. D. FORM NO. 18b (STATEMENT OF EXPENDITURE OF SPECIAL DENTAL MATERIALS)

	Paragraph
Where required	211
System of weights used	212
Preparation	213

211. Where required.—This report is required from every military station or separate command where a dental clinic with laboratory facilities is established and a dental officer is in attendance. It will be forwarded monthly in accordance with circular letter No. 61, S. G. O., June 16, 1941.

212. **System of weights used.**—To understand this form one must first be familiar with the system of weights used in weighing gold. This system differs from the decimal system which is used in the accounting of funds, and therefore at first presents some difficulties. The scale used is as follows:

$$24 \text{ grains} = 1 \text{ pennyweight.}$$
$$20 \text{ pennyweight} = 1 \text{ ounce.}$$

Form No. 18b makes provision for recording only pennyweight (dwt) and grains (gr).

213. **Preparation.**—*a. Heading.*—The name of the station is entered on the top of the report preceded by the code number of the station. Code numbers have been assigned to all stations by the Chief of Finance. These numbers will precede the names of the stations on all papers pertaining to medical supplies (that is, 429—Fort Jay, N. Y.).

b. Paragraph 1.—Enter the following under paragraph 1: name, grade, organization, nature of appliance, amount of gold used, and date of insertion of all appliances (for military personnel). In the description of the appliance, first the teeth replaced or repaired are entered (including surfaces involved for inlays); then the appliance constructed using authorized abbreviations. Examples: R4, mod Inlay, gold; R13, 14, 15, L13, 14, 15. Dtr. Pr. C/3 B/1.

c. Paragraph 2.—Under paragraph 2 the same is accomplished for others entitled to treatment.

d. Paragraph 3.—In paragraph 3, statement of materials, amounts of special materials on hand last report, amounts received, amounts expended, and amounts remaining on hand at close of period will be entered together with such explanatory remarks as may be necessary. The report will be signed by the dental officer immediately responsible for the special dental materials.

e. Computing weights.—In adding the columns of pennyweights (dwt) and grains (gr), it must be remembered to treat these columns separately. First, the grains column is added and the total is divided by 24. This will give the pennyweight and the remainder will be the number of grains. The remainder is entered as the grains total and the whole number is added in the pennyweight (dwt) column. One must keep in mind when computing or checking this report that he is not dealing with the decimal system and that 24 grains equal 1 pennyweight.

Section V

DAILY WORK SHEET

Paragraph
Preparation_____ 214

214. Preparation.—The daily work sheet is not an officially designated dental record and no Medical Department form is furnished for its preparation. It is, however, a very important record and some form of work sheet is of great value. This record is made out at the chair at the completion of each sitting and serves as a temporary record from which Form No. 79 is made, and a permanent, easily tabulated record of work performed by each officer for any given period. A very satisfactory work sheet can be made locally, either mimeographed or printed on 8- by 13-inch paper. Lines should extend the length of the paper to form a space for each patient. Lines across the paper should divide it into columns for name, Army serial number, grade, organization, age, State of birth, length of service, diagnosis, treatment, and classification. These data should be complete on all new admissions and in addition should show whether the patient is a routine or emergency admission. At subsequent sittings only sufficient personal data to identify the patient's card are necessary, but a complete diagnosis of conditions treated and operations performed must be entered at each sitting. The data to fill out and complete Form No. 79 are taken from the daily work sheet, hence it is very essential that all entries are comprehensive and complete.

Section VI

HOSPITAL CLINIC RECORDS

Paragraph
General_____ 215
Forms used_____ 216
W. D., M. D. Form No. 55E-4 (Clinical Record, Dental Examination)_____ 217
W. D., M. D. Form No. 55E-5 (Clinical Record, Dental Record)_____ 218
Other forms_____ 219

215. General.—The clinical records of patients in military hospitals are probably the most important records for which the Medical Department of the Army is responsible. In addition to furnishing a valuable source from which statistical data may be obtained, they often form the basis for claims against the Government and other similar actions. For the protection of both the Government and the individual concerned, if for no other reasons, clinical records should be complete and accurate.

216. Forms used.—The new clinical record forms are on typewriter size paper and compose a group of about 33 forms. Of these, W. D., M. D. Forms Nos. 55E–4 and 55E–5 are the dental forms. Every sheet of the clinical record must be authenticated by the officer preparing it. The first entry made in the record by any officer must be signed; subsequent entries may be initialed. The component parts of the clinical record are kept in the chart holder and in the correct order. The chart holder is kept in the ward office on the ward to which the patient is assigned. The clinical record should not be entrusted to the patient for delivery from one department or ward to another, nor should patients be allowed to read them.

217. W. D., M. D. Form No. 55E–4 (Clinical Record, Dental Examination).—This form is a combined request for a report of a special examination and the finished report of that examination. The ward surgeon uses the top part of the front page of this form to refer patients to the dental clinic. The form is so arranged that the ward surgeon may indicate whether the patient has been referred for emergency or routine treatment, the elimination of dental foci, or for only examination and report and no treatment. This form may also be used to notify the dental service that a patient has been admitted for dental treatment only. The reverse side of this form is used by the dental officer when conducting his examination. The chart should be filled out using the key to indicate the conditions noted. All the findings or diagnoses determined as a result of the dental examination should be recorded in the order of their importance on the lower half of the front page. The form is then returned to the ward and becomes a part of the patient's clinical record. In the event that a definite diagnosis cannot be determined immediately, this form should be returned to the ward with a tentative diagnosis and a list of the laboratory tests, consultations, and other diagnostic procedures contemplated.

218. W. D., M. D. Form No. 55E–5 (Clinical Record, Dental Record).—This form is prepared by the dental service; a duplicate of Form No. 79 was formerly used for this purpose. It should contain a summary of the treatment rendered by the dental service together with the final diagnosis. In the cases where foci have been eliminated, the form is to be prepared in duplicate. The ward officer notes any improvement in the condition of the patient as a result of treatment and returns one copy to the dental service. The data so obtained are used to compile statistics.

219. Other forms.—When the patient is hospitalized primarily for a dental condition, the dental officer will be responsible for more of the clinical record than the two purely dental forms mentioned above. However, the record clerk, dental service, will not have to assist in preparing any other forms except Forms Nos. 55E-4 and 55E-5.

Section VII

W. D., A. G. O. FORMS

	Paragraph
W. D., A. G. O. Form No. 63 (Report of Physical Examination)	220
W. D., A. G. O. Form No. 258 (Physical Record)	221

220. W. D., A. G. O. Form No. 63 (Report of Physical Examination).—This form contains a section for dental examination. A chart of the teeth appears on this form, and a restorable carious tooth is marked by a circle around the number representing that tooth; a nonrestorable carious tooth is marked by a diagonal line; and a missing tooth is indicated by an X through the number representing the tooth. Bridges and dentures may be indicated on the chart by the symbols illustrated on the reverse side of W. D., M. D. Form No. 79.

221. W. D., A. G. O. Form No. 258 (Physical Record).—This is a form which is filed with the enlisted man's service record, but it should be brought to the dental clinic when the enlisted man reports for dental attendance. All routine dental operations and treatments must be recorded briefly on this form; it must be signed and dated by the dental officer. Abbreviations authorized in AR 40-1010 may be used on this form, and all dental operations should be described thereon as briefly as possible.

Section VIII

DENTAL SURVEY

	Paragraph
Purpose	222
Procedure	223
Use	224

222. Purpose.—The dental survey, the record of which is described in section I, is the process by which the dental efficiency of the group is determined. It serves for the group as does the dental examination for the individual. By a study of the record of the dental survey, it is possible to make an accurate estimate of the dental needs of the command. It is the basis upon which the dental officer determines those who should receive treatment and the priority in which they should receive it. It is for this reason an essential preliminary step to the institution of dental service for any command. The consolidated results of a dental survey represent the estimate of the dental situation which must be met by the dental service.

223. Procedure.—Dental officers serving with troops will sometimes find that much time can be saved by surveying organizations in places other than the dental office. Generally the following procedure is followed:

a. The organizations report at a designated place with two copies of pay roll roster on 8- by 10½-inch standard letter paper, which lists the grade, name, age, place of birth, and years of service of every man in the organization.

b. The officer or noncommissioned officer in charge will form the men in single file as their names appear on the roster.

c. A noncommissioned officer who knows most of the men in the organization by name will act as clerk during the survey. He is instructed to place the classification (I, II, III, or IV) before each man's name as the dental officer indicates. Sometimes the surveying officer prefers to indicate relative urgency in a given classification by adding the symbols plus or double plus as the case may be.

d. The dental officer stations himself with the enlisted assistant at a selected spot with the light, artificial or natural, coming from behind.

e. A sufficient supply of wooden tongue depressors, mouth mirrors, explorers, and suitable means for sterilizing the mirrors and explorers in use is provided.

f. Each man steps up before the dental officer and opens his mouth. The dental officer, usually with only the use of a tongue depressor, examines the mouth and indicates the classification of the individual to the clerk.

g. At the conclusion of the survey, the dental officer directs the noncommissioned officer acting as clerk to make a list of all absentees. It is arranged to have these report to the dental office at a designated time.

224. Use.—The completed dental survey is entrusted to the record clerk in the dental office who uses it to obtain data for the reports. The record clerk is responsible for changing the classification on the survey as the men come to the clinic for treatment.

Section IX

DENTAL HISTORY OF STATION

	Paragraph
General	225
Composition	226
Filing	227

225. General.—Regulations require that a dental history be maintained at each station in the zone of the interior where a dental officer is on duty. The compiling and filing of this record will be one of the duties of the record clerk.

226. Composition.—The dental history will consist of the retained copies of the reports and records (W. D., M. D. Forms Nos. 57 and 18b) together with the following:

a. Reports of dental opinions on clinics.

b. Schedules of instruction for enlisted assistants.

c. Memoranda recommended for incorporation in sanitary orders.

d. Special reports and articles for publication.

e. Such other data as are deemed pertinent.

227. Filing.—At the close of each month and upon completion of all reports required for the month, the retained copies of the reports will be filed, fastened together as "Dental History, Fort ——————, for the month of ——————". At the close of each calendar year an index of all items mentioned in the preceding paragraphs will be prepared and filed as an index to the dental history for that year.

APPENDIX

LIST OF REFERENCES

"Dental Anatomy"—Black, G. V. Philadelphia: S. S. White Co., 1897.

"Dental Anatomy"—Diamond, M. New York: MacMillan Co., 1935.

"Practical Dental Anatomy and Tooth Carving"—Schwartz, J. R. Brooklyn: Dental Items of Interest Publishing Co., 1935.

INDEX

	Paragraph	Page
Acrylic resin:		
Dentures	49	59
Repair	58	66
Splints	96	98
Use	50	59
Adjustable articulators	11	14
Air compressor	190	164
Alloy	15	18
Alveolar process	15, 140	18, 137
Alveolus	15	18
Amalgam:		
Copper	197	169
Silver	196	169
Anatomy, regional	8–14	10
Anesthetic solution	193	167
Angles in X-ray technique	104, 105	106, 108
Apex, root	15	18
Apical foramina	140	137
Appointments	192	166
Apthous stomatitis	149	142
Areas, relief in dentures	27	29
Articulation, temporomandibular	11	14
Articulators	11	14
Assembling plaster impressions	19	24
Atrophy of gingivae	153	142
Autoclave	177	159
Axial surfaces	15	18
Bacilli	176	158
Bacteria	176	158
Bacteriology of sterilization	176	158
Band crown	66	72
Bars:		
For partial dentures	72–78	80
Lingual and palatal	78	86
Bell crowned	15	18
Bismuth stomatitis	150	142
Biteplates	29	32
Boxing impressions	20, 24	25, 27
Bridge, fixed	68–71	75
Buccal surface	6	8

INDEX

	Paragraph	Page
Buccinator muscle	142	139
Burs	185	163
Calculus	156	143
Care:		
Dental clinic	173, 174	156, 157
Mouth and teeth	168–170	152
Caries	143, 144	139, 140
Cartridge-type syringe	193	167
Cast clasps	77	85
Casting:		
Dental	59–62	66
Investment	62	67
Partial dentures	93	95
Cast occlusal crown	66	72
Casts:		
Mounting on articulator	30	33
Partial dentures	79	87
Pouring	21	26
Separation	22, 25	26, 28
Cement	198	169
Cementum	15, 140	18, 137
Chair assistant	171, 172	155, 156
Clasp:		
Cast	77	85
Crib	76	85
For partial dentures	72–78	80
Repair of loose	54	64
Wrought	73	82
Classification of patients	206	175
Cleft palate	3	5
Clinic, care and cleaning	173–174	156
Cocci	176	158
Compound impressions	23	27
Contact point	15	18
Copper amalgam	197	169
Cresol	178	159
Crib clasp	76	85
Crown:		
Band	66	72
Cast	63–65	71
Die	64	71
Three-quarter	63	71
Crown and bridge cement	198	169
Cusp	15	18
Cutting edge	15	18
Daily work sheet	218	187
Darkroom, X-ray	131	131

INDEX

	Paragraph	Page
Deciduous teeth	15	18
Dental—		
Burs	185	163
Caries	143	139
Engine	186	163
Floss	164	150
History	225–227	190
Hygiene	139	137
Hygienist	139	137
Lathe	188	164
Survey	222	188
Dentine	15, 140	18, 137
Denture:		
Acrylic resin	49	59
Base, trial	28	30
Duplicating	57	65
Flasking	44, 45	52, 53
Polishing	48	58
Rebasing	56	65
Refacing	55	64
Repair	51–58	62
Waxing	43	51
Depressor muscles	142	139
Designing partial denture	81	88
Digastric muscle	142	139
Disclosing solution	165	150
Diseases of mouth	145–153	141
Distal surface	6	8
Embrasure	15	18
Enamel	15	18
Engine and handpiece	186	163
Equipment, care	182	161
Eugenol	200	171
External pterygoid muscle	12, 142	16, 139
Extra-oral roentgenography	126–129	125
Facial	15	18
Facial surface	6	8
Filling materials	195	168
Films, X-ray	100	103
Fissure	15	18
Fixed bridge	68–71	75
Flasking	44–45	52
Floss, dental	164	150
Foramen:		
Anterior palatal	9	11
Definition	15	18
Posterior palatal	9	11

INDEX

	Paragraph	Page
Formina. *See* Foramen.		
Forceps, care	187	164
Forms:		
A. G. O.:		
63	220	188
258	221	188
Medical Department:		
16a, b, c, d	203	174
18b	211–213	184
55E–4 and 55E–5	216	187
57	206, 207	175, 179
65	203	174
79	208–210	183
Fossa	15	18
Frenum:		
Labium inferioris	13	17
Labium superioris	13	17
Linguae	13	17
Gargle	170	153
Genioglossus	142	139
Geniohyoid muscle	142	139
Gingiva	15, 140	18, 137
Gingival—		
Atrophy	153	142
Line	15	18
Margin	140	137
Gingivitis	151, 152	142
Glenoid fossa	11	14
Gold:		
Heat treatment	75	84
Report	211	184
Green stain	157	143
Groove	15	18
Gum	140	137
Hand instruments	184	162
Handling patients	192	166
Handpiece	186	163
Heat treatment, gold	75	84
History, dental	225–227	190
Hospital clinic records	215–219	186
Hydrocolloid impressions	26	28
Hygiene	139	137
Hypertrophic gingivitis	152	142
Hypodermic syringes	180	160
Impression:		
Boxing	20	25
Hydrocolloid	26	28
Materials	17, 194	23, 168

INDEX

	Paragraph	Page
Incisal surface	6	8
Inclination	15	18
Instrumentation	160	145
Instruments	158, 184	144, 162
Intensifying screen	103	105
Internal pterygoid muscle	12, 142	16, 139
Interproximal embrasure	15	18
Interproximal space	15	18
Intra-oral X-rays	104–125	106
Investing, partial denture pattern	92	95
Kilovoltage, in X-ray	102	104
Labial surface	6	8
Lathe	188	164
Lingual—		
Bars	78	86
Surface	6	8
Lysol	178	159
Malocclusion	141	138
Mandible	10	13
Marginal ridge	15	18
Massage of gums	167	152
Masseter muscle	12, 142	16, 139
Mastication	142	139
Median line	5, 15	7, 18
Medicaments	183	161
Mesial surface	6	8
Microbe	176	158
Milliamperage, in X-ray	102	104
Mirror, mouth	158	144
Model, duplication	87	92
Modeling compound impressions	23–25	27
Monthly reports	206	175
Mounting casts on articulator	30	33
Mouth	2–15	4
Mirror	158	144
Mouthwash	170	153
Mucin	155	143
Mucous membrane	3	5
Muscles	12, 142	16, 139
Neck, tooth	15	18
Needles, hypodermic	180	160
Nerve, tooth	140	137
Oblique ridge	15	18
Occlusal:		
Rests	74	83
Surface	6	8

INDEX

	Paragraph	Page
Occlusion	141	138
Oxyphosphate cement	198	169
Packing the case	46	54
Palate	3, 9	5, 11
Paradentosis	146	141
Partial denture:		
Cast	79	87
Casting	93	95
Design	81	88
Flasking	45	53
Investing	92	95
Spruing	91	94
Waxing	90	93
Periodontal diseases	145	141
Periodontoclasia	146	141
Personal hygiene	172	156
Physical record	221	188
Physiology, mouth and teeth	140–142	137
Pickling	62	67
Pit	15	18
Plaster impressions	18–22	24
Platysma muscle	142	139
Polishing, oral hygiene	163	149
Porcelain, synthetic	199	170
Pouring of casts	21	26
Precautions, in X-ray	102	104
Processing X-ray films	130–138	131
Prophylaxis	158–161	144
Prosthetic dentistry	16	22
Prosthodontia	16	22
Protozoa	176	158
Proximal surface	15	18
Pulp	140	137
Raphe, palatal	9	11
Rebasing dentures	56	65
Refacing dentures	55	64
Regional anatomy	8–14	10
Register of dental patients	208–210	183
Relief areas	27	29
Report:		
Dental service	206, 207	175, 179
Physical examination	224	189
Root canal	140	137
Routine, clinical	201	171
Rubber packing	46	54
Rugae	9	11
Rules of sterlization	178	159

INDEX

	Paragraph	Page
Saliva	142, 154	139, 142
Sanitation	181	160
Scalers	158	144
Separation of casts	22	26
Septum	15	18
Silicate	199	170
Silver splints	97	99
Slab, care	187	164
Solutions, X-ray	137	132
Splints	94–97	96
Stain	157	143
Staphylococcus	176	158
Statement of expenditure of special dental materials	211–213	184
Sterilization	175–181	158
Sterilizers	177	159
Stomatitis	148–150	141
Streptococcus	176	158
Structure, mouth	3	5
Styloglossus	142	139
Sulcus	15	18
Supplemental groove and ridge	15	18
Supplies, care	182	161
Survey, dental	222–224	188
Surveying model	82	89
Synthetic porcelain	199	170
Syringes, hypodermic	180, 193	160, 167
Systemic cause of caries	144	140
Tartar	156	143
Teeth:		
Added to denture	53	64
Arranging	33–41	36
Arranging upper anteriors	33	36
Artificial, selection	31	35
Broken or loose on dentures	52	63
Central dental laboratory assortment	42	48
Classification	4	7
Loose, in dentures	52	63
Roots	7	9
Setting up	33–41	36
Structure	140	137
Surfaces	6	8
System of naming and numbering	5	7
Telephone calls	192	166
Temporal muscle	12, 142	16, 139
Temporomandibular roentgenography	128	127
Tongue muscles	142	139
Tooth:		
Brushing method	166	151
Forms	32	35

INDEX

	Paragraph	Page
Tooth—Continued.		
Nerve	140	137
Paste	169	153
Powders	169	153
Torus palatinus	14	18
Transverse ridge	15	18
Trial denture base	28	30
Tripoding	86	91
Trubyte teeth	42	48
Tubercle	15	18
Uvula	3	5
Vincent's stomatitis	148	141
Voltage in X-ray	102	104
Vulcanite splints	95	96
Vulcanization	47	57
Vulcanizer	189	164
Wax pattern	60, 61	67
Waxing	43, 90	51, 93
Wrought clasps	73	82
X-ray:		
Bite wing	107	110
Darkroom	131	131
Extra-oral	126–129	125
Films	100	103
Intra-oral	104–125	106
Machine	99	103
Occlusal	119	120
Physics	102	104
Processing	130–138	131
Solutions	137	132
Temporomandibular joint	128	127
Zinc oxide	200	171

[A. G. 062.11 (10–7–41).]

By order of the Secretary of War:

                                G. C. MARSHALL,
                                    Chief of Staff.

Official:
    E. S. ADAMS,
        Major General,
            The Adjutant General.

Distribution:
    X.
    (For explanation of symbols see FM 21–6.)